Fly Fishi Sharks:

A memoir of life with OCD

To Adrian

To one who knows.

Andrew.

Andrew Alexander

Andrew Alexander

Published by
Chipmunkapublishing
PO Box 6872
Brentwood
Essex CM13 1ZT
United Kingdom

http://www.chipmunkapublishing.com

Fly Fishing For Sharks

CONTENTS
Prologue

Andrew Alexander

Fly Fishing For Sharks

Prologue

I am thirty-two. I haven't bedded any famous women or travelled to exotic locations, triumphed over poverty or fought in a war. I am currently unemployed and have been for a decent chunk of my twenties. I live with my parents, my hair is thinning and my curriculum vitae is getting worse by the minute. So what makes me think I should write an autobiography?

I started writing this book because I was angry. I knew that if I didn't do something constructive with my anger, I would end up doing something utterly irrational that would have long-term consequences. I had been out running one evening and was running against the traffic which, as every runner knows, is safer because you can spot any errant vehicles as they approach and take evasive action. I was gesticulating at the oncoming traffic so they would give me a wide enough berth. Most of them complied, but there was one truck that came too close.

I stopped, turned around and began to swear hysterically and aim both middle fingers at his rear-view mirror. I'm sure he was unaware of my tirade but, as a worried mother covered her child's ears in a nearby driveway, it struck me that I was poisoning myself with anger and bitterness and that something must be done.

Do I have a right to be angry and bitter? I would like you to be the judge of that but you are going to have to read this book first. I have never written a book before and I don't consider myself much of a writer, but I think I have a story to tell that you might find interesting. In addition, it would be dishonest of me not to admit that I am looking for validation. I seek validation because, from an economic and financial perspective, I feel like redundant machinery for which spare parts are no longer available. When you don't have a job, you don't feel very good about yourself and when you haven't worked for long stretches of your adulthood, worse.

I read somewhere that the suicide rate for unemployed adult males is fifteen to twenty times higher than in the normal population. I am not surprised. I think it was Henry Kissinger who said that power is the ultimate aphrodisiac. Well, unemployment is the ultimate turn-off. And not having a healthy sex life is a recipe for glumness and despondency. Some religious folks opt to abstain from intercourse in the quest for spiritual intimacy with God, but for most of us, abstinence is going a bit too far.

This book is about my battle with Obsessive-Compulsive Disorder – from here on in I will use the acronym OCD. I hope to make it a good read for those who don't have the disorder and a source of solace for those who do.

The entertainment industry has given us, as far as I am aware, three portrayals of OCD. There was the movie, *As Good As It Gets*, with Jack Nicholson; and I have seen a few episodes of a series called *Monk* about a detective with OCD. Both these offerings portrayed largely functional OCD sufferers. Jack Nicholson was a successful, although slightly irascible, writer; and Monk seemed to be gainfully employed as a solver of crimes. This is not my experience of OCD. In *The Aviator*, a film about the life of Howard Hughes, an obsession with germs and contamination sometimes reduced Leonardo DiCaprio's character to an existence of self-imposed hermetic isolation. Despite being a brilliant and immensely successful man, Hughes spent his last days in the grip of his contamination obsession. I can relate more to Howard Hughes than Jack Nicholson's character or Monk, although it must be added that Howard's success is not mirrored in these pages.

In my case, OCD dragged me into a world of terror, Clinical Depression and desperation that resulted in suicide attempts and admissions to psychiatric hospitals. It transformed me from a confident teenager into an adult who felt so overwhelmed by life that I was intimidated by the act of showering.

I have also been very lucky through it all. I have parents who can afford the expense of treatment; and friends who have stood by me during the worst times. I have had periods of functionality and happiness and have experienced the delights of falling in love. I know that things could have been worse and that others are suffering in ways that I can only imagine.

However, the varying severity of suffering experienced by others should never be used to manipulate people into feeling that they don't have a right to grieve over what life has taken from them. We all have different capacities for suffering and, as such, an emotionally resilient person might withstand a trauma that would devastate someone who is more fragile.

I once worked for a man who had kindly created a position for me in his company. After a couple of months I felt that I was not coping with the job and was starting to spiral down into Depression as a result. I resigned and on my last day at the job my boss said to me, "You know, other people have much worse problems than you and they soldier on."

He was right. But it was one of the most insensitive things anyone has ever said to me because he was trying to minimise what I had gone through and belittle the progress I had made. Be wary of confiding in the large majority of the confident and successful because their egos tend to retard their ability to empathise. You will have to excuse the odd sardonic aphorism - it is all part of the healing process.

A footnote: When it comes to personal pronouns, the gender-sensitive approach is to use 'he or she'. I find this cumbersome, although I agree with being gender sensitive, and so I flipped a coin – heads was for he, tails was for she. It came up heads.

Chapter I

You dirty little boy

I was born in Cape Town, South Africa in March 1976, a few months before the Soweto uprisings inflamed the nation and the tide started to turn on *apartheid*. My parents had met and fallen in love while at university in Cape Town; and when they completed their studies, they married and settled in a little house by the sea about half an hour's drive from the city. It was idyllic, with the beach as my playground and two doting parents hanging on my every gurgle.

But all was not well in the Republic of South Africa as the elaborate idiocy that was *apartheid* began to look economically unsustainable and increasingly ideologically indefensible in the international community. In 1980 my parents moved the family back to their native Zimbabwe after the birth of my sister. My mother was a progressive woman who didn't want her children educated in a country where they would be accorded special privileges because they were white. In addition, Zimbabwe achieved independence in 1980 and the new President, Robert Mugabe, spoke of reconciliation and forgiveness in his inaugural address to the nation. This informed our move but was later to prove a naïve premise on which to emigrate. However, our extended family lived in Zimbabwe and the schooling was based on the British system. My siblings and I were thus likely to get a better education than in South Africa.

Zimbabwe was a fine country in which to be a child. The climate in Harare is so pleasant that you tend to become irritated at the slightest hint of inclement weather; and if it lasts more than a day or two, people go into decline. If you were even vaguely middle class you could afford a large house, a big garden and perhaps even a pool. What made parenting such a pleasure was the cost of domestic help. Many very average families had at least one, if not two, employees and some had three or four. This was all to do with the distortions of colonialism that were a feature of Zimbabwean society even after independence.

My only hassle was my damn lips. I had a Swedish grandfather from whom I inherited a limited tolerance for ultraviolet light. Harare is in the tropics where the sunlight is very strong. I would frequently end a day in the sun with blisters on my lips which turned into bloody scabs within a day or two. All this despite the assiduous application of RayStop – Zimbabwe's locally made and utterly useless brand of sunscreen. Despite legions of unfortunate white settlers who developed skin cancer as the years went by, Zimbabwe's cosmetics giants never churned out much in the way of sunscreen and we were forced to rely on overseas visitors to provide the real thing.

Suffice it to say, I had a happy childhood without any obvious trauma. I mention this because one of my psychiatrists spent a vast amount of time looking for the source of my illness in childhood experiences. He showed an inordinate interest in the strictness of my potty training. The problem was, I had absolutely no recollection of my potty training. I think this was one of Freud's insights, developed before we knew much about brain chemistry and genetic predispositions. I shudder to think of those poor OCD sufferers in times gone by who paid good money in the hope of getting some relief from their symptoms, only to be told that their salvation lay in the in-depth analysis of their long-forgotten experiences of learning to defecate and urinate in a socially acceptable manner. Freud might have been right but my psychiatrist may as well have asked me if breast milk was an acquired taste or something I liked immediately.

There *is* something in my childhood that might be relevant to the OCD that developed later. Childhood sexuality is an emotive topic but it is a fact of life and a normal part of growing up. As I write this, countless games of Doctor-Doctor are going on around the world as children explore each other's anatomies and, alas, countless parents are finding out and overreacting.

I think I learnt about sex when I was about eight. I was at a friend's house and his older brother and one of his friends took us to the bottom of the garden, sat us down and told us the ins and outs – sorry, couldn't resist that one. I remember feeling a bit baffled about what to do with this information; and also a vague sense of being dirty for knowing these things. I am not sure what their motives were but I assume they were simply new to adolescence and not sure how to process their own sexual awakening. Much like a born-again Christian in the early phases of their conversion, they were just spreading the good news. I think my friend and I just walked away and continued constructing various structures out of Lego.

I'm not sure when the first sex games happened but it was sometime over the following two years. I was involved but I don't remember actually initiating it. It happened at our house and involved a girl and some of my friends. There was no coercion or actual penetration but we knew what we were simulating. We took it in turns to lie on top of the girl and then, with the aid of the other protagonists, we would roll over a few times. That was it.

I remember another incident when I persuaded a girl I knew to take off her clothes and dance for some other children. It happened at our house and I felt responsible for the entertainment. This was before Cartoon Network and video games. I do feel that I asked a bit too much from that poor girl, but if we are going to judge actions on their consequences, I think it was pretty harmless. She went on to have a successful career and a happy marriage – and no, it wasn't as a stripper.

In August 1986, on a brilliant blue Saturday morning, my father called me aside and said he wanted to talk about something. He took me into my room and he seemed angry. I remember sitting on my bed looking up at his looming adult frame and knowing that I was in trouble. He started telling me that some parents had phoned asking for details about the games we were playing and I remember clearly him saying that they were angry. In my mind I imagined them to be hysterically angry, the kind of anger that seeks to destroy the object of opprobrium. It transpired that even a teacher at school knew what had happened. Something in the tone of my father's voice implied that what had happened was disgraceful and shameful and that the community at large was outraged. Worse still, I inferred from what he said that I was considered the ringleader and was being singled out for most of the blame.

Adult sexual neurosis had been applied to pre-pubescent exploration and, because I was a child who didn't know any better, I was thrust into the adult world of hypocrisy and guilt. I felt a surge of shame. I started crying and denied any knowledge of what my father was referring to. He kept asking about the games and I continued to sob. When my father saw that he was getting nowhere, he let me go. I remember walking outside into the sunlight and feeling the contrast between the warmth of the sun and cold stab of shame piercing my conscience.

Other fathers might have beaten their sons. Perhaps if I had been beaten there would have been some kind of catharsis as the pain of the punishment matched the pain of the guilt. I simply don't know. But I carried that guilt for years and with it, a deep sense that I deserved punishment of some kind.

Chapter II

Deuteronomy for the horny teenager

If childhood sexuality is a touchy subject, discussing religion is just asking for trouble. But it must be done.

I had grown up in a nominally Christian environment because my mom was a convert. She was admirably balanced about the whole thing and never attempted any indoctrination. I remember singing hymns at school and being quite fond of 'Amazing Grace', but not having any sense of salvation, afterlife or a personal relationship with God. As a family, we went occasionally to an Anglican church where, after the singing, the children were shipped off to Sunday School for more singing and Bible stories. It didn't make much of an impression on me. I remember a slight aversion to the name 'Sunday School' because I felt that I already spent five days a week at school and, even at that early age, I considered the weekend to be a time of leisure and frivolity, notwithstanding the fact that I was one of father Abraham's many sons.

I once went with a friend to a charismatic church that his mother attended. It was held in a huge hall and the singing was considerably more animated than at the Anglican Church. People stood on chairs and danced in the aisles and the pastor had the manic energy of a motivational speaker. When he prayed between songs there was much support from the congregation in as much as when he said something really spiritual, ripples of "Amen!", "Hallelujah!" and "Thank you, Jesus!" spread out along the pews. My friend and I were sent off to Sunday School after the singing and that was when I had my first experience of speaking in tongues.

Fly Fishing For Sharks

For Christians, speaking in tongues is cool. According to the Bible it is a gift that certain people have or, rather, are given. This church was having none of that and was keen to give all the young members a head start in the tongues game. So, with minimal instruction, we were encouraged to just give it a go.

The important thing with tongues is that it must be unintelligible to the listener so actual words are not to be uttered. Unfortunately, there are a limited number of entirely novel sounds that the average human can produce in a continuous stream. The result is some sort of vaguely repeating pattern from the less gifted and utter gibberish from the more inventive. I think I said some version of "shubalamalakalashubalamalaka" over and over until the youth pastor told us we could stop.

Years later I was in a church service during which a member of the congregation stood up and announced that she had received a message from above. She then spoke for a couple of minutes in tongues and sat down. The pastor asked if anyone had received the translation for the message. "This is going to be good," I thought. Sure enough, a brave guy stood up and declared that he had decoded the message. With an astrologer's gift for vagueness and ambiguity he told us what the tongues had meant. People were impressed and the service went on. Although I was a believer at the time, it occurred to me that a *Tongues Phrasebook* would not go amiss for those of us who didn't have the privilege of receiving divine translation.

My approach to religion changed drastically one Saturday afternoon when I was twelve. I was having an afternoon lie down at a friend's house and I was bored, so I got up and perused the bookshelf. I can't remember what the book was called but it was a book for children explaining Christianity.

I remember the last page. It depicted Judgement Day and showed God in a chair sending some people up to heaven and some people down to hell, which was shown in the picture as a fire. The accompanying text explained that Christians go to Heaven and unbelievers and sinners go to hell where, according to the picture, they burn.

Whatever a twelve-year-old would have said in those days instead of, "Oh fuck," I said it. The horrible thing is that that book was conceived and written by adults. Surely there is a better way to introduce children to what, after all, is supposed to be a message of love, than to scare the living daylights out of them? For a kid who plays sex games and occasionally raids the family milk money to splurge at the tuck shop, it seemed to me that the flames of hell beckoned. I concluded that Christianity was the only option.

I approached my mother and asked her how I could become a Christian. She explained the basic principles of conversion and a few weeks later I was up at the front of the Church asking God to come into my life. I prayed for forgiveness, then the pastor prayed on my behalf, and that was it. I was northbound out of Hades.

A few of the most wonderful people that I have met are Christians and I have a great respect for some people of faith. In truth, it is not their faith that I respect, but rather their attempts to alleviate suffering. Having said that, some of the most bigoted and ignorant people I have met have also been Christians. They tend to be Christian fundamentalists who sanctify their intolerance by claiming it is mandated by their faith. A secular bigot will say, "I hate faggots because what they do is disgusting." A religious bigot will say, "Homosexuality is an abomination in the eyes of God. I can love the sinner but never the sin." The second statement is worse than the first because it is manipulative as well as bigoted. Separating sexual orientation from identity and labelling it unworthy of love is patronising and cruel. What the religious bigot is really saying is, "I'm glad God hates the same thing as me because now I can hold onto my prejudice and please God at the same time."

There has to be a more loving way to attract converts than to say "the wages of sin is death" or, more crudely, "turn or burn". Of course people are going to give their lives to the Lord if they are scared shitless of going to hell, especially people with anxiety disorders like me.

Childhood was an uncomplicated time to be a Christian. I think I was reasonably well behaved and quite diligent at school and my sins were relatively minor. It was also a massive relief to know that God was a forgiveness kind of guy: you just had to ask and say sorry - and mean it of course.

Adolescence changed everything. It brought a new sin – masturbation. The word even sounds dirty. It seems linguistically crafted to induce guilt. I discovered it on my own without knowing what an orgasm or sperm was. It was August 1989 and boy was I glad to be alive. I was staggered that anything could feel so good, and for the first couple of months I would dart off to the bathroom as soon as I felt horny and vigorously debunk the notion that there is no such thing as a free lunch.

The first year after my discovery was a period of spirited and guilt-free jerking-off. Initially it was enough to just tug away, but then I discovered to my delight that you could enhance the experience by creating elaborate fantasies. An orgasm was powerfully enhanced by the mental image that you were doing whatever it takes to make the most beautiful girl in town moan with ecstasy, while her equally sexy best friend lay naked and wanton on the other side of the double bed, seductively beckoning you with gloriously implausible phrases of uninhibited lust. That freedom to roam the fecund plains of sexual possibility is a tribute to the power of the mind.

There was an organisation in Harare that ran Christian camps for teenage boys during the school holidays. The guy who ran them was an avuncular fellow who did a service to his community by keeping plenty of boys out of mischief by preaching clean living and an outdoor lifestyle of activity and fun. He had one quirk that, as quirks go, was odder than most. He seemed to think that boys should feel comfortable about their naked bodies and, to this end, he instituted some mildly unsettling practices into camp life. For example, we were asked to leave our towels in the shower room, which meant we had to walk to and from our dormitories in the nude twice a day. This was problematic in the morning because most teenage boys wake up with a raging erection that needs time to settle.

Deuteronomy, for want of a better pseudonym, would stride through the dormitories naked, with a towel draped over his shoulder and a certain urgency in his voice, informing us that it was, "Shower time, men." We used to joke about how bizarre it was to open your eyes and see a middle-aged set of reproductive equipment only a few feet away. Knowing that your towel was in the showers meant that you had about half a minute to suppress your erection before suffering the indignity of walking to the showers in full bloom. Every morning we would lie there thinking of the least erotic thing we could possibly imagine in order to affect the necessary detumescence.

One of the aims of these camps was to provide a fun environment for saving souls. There were compulsory meetings each evening that featured the singing of catchy songs and then a short talk, usually by Deuteronomy. The first three nights were devoted to the usual conversion tactics. On night one, you were told that all had sinned and fallen short of the glory of God - I think most people thought that was basically true. Night two, you were hit with the big one: the wages of sin is death. On night three, Deuteronomy smiled kindly at the audience and offered the ticket to salvation: give your life to Jesus and accept his offer of eternity in heaven. At the end of night four's meeting, Deuteronomy announced that anyone who wanted to become a Christian should present himself at the front of the hall to receive Christ into his heart.

The camp was divided into three groups. Group one were already Christian, as I was, and felt secure. Group two were those brave souls who weren't buying any of it. Group three were in a muddle. "Oh shit – wait, is that a sin? I mean, oh shuttlecock – no, not cock, that's rude. Oh heck, I'm going to hell." Group one got very excited about all the new converts responding to the altar call. Group two was thinking, "Maybe I should have asked my parents for a new bike rather than getting them to pay good money for this circus,"; or they saw one of their friends going to the front and were pissed off because they would now have to find another drinking buddy. Group three was slowly making its way to the front of the hall, torn between the desire to avoid being paid the wages of sin at some later date and the need to save face with the predominantly alpha males in group two who looked on disapprovingly.

Day five dawned bright and still. That evening Deuteronomy gave a talk entitled 'Wine, Women and Song'. I didn't drink at the time and so wholeheartedly concurred with the strong warnings about the dangers of alcohol. I was a little surprised by Deuteronomy's claims that a lot of the songs I enjoyed were anti-Christian and deeply immoral. I found out that the band AC/DC meant 'anti-Christ, devil's children'. This meant that I had to pretend that I wasn't electrified to my core by the song *Thunderstruck*. Deuteronomy said that the expression 'Rock'n'Roll' actually meant having sex in a moving car.

He then moved onto women. According to this arbiter of sexual norms and customs, an erection was a warning light that things had gone too far with your date. I was in grave trouble because I got erections at female swimming galas and I wasn't within ten feet of a woman. I don't think I'm a good-looking fellow and so it was still years before I had to face the dilemma of how far to go with a date, by which time I was well into adulthood. Deuteronomy emphasised that premarital sex was to be avoided at all costs and added that warning lights were helpful to this end. I think that when it comes to premarital sex, heaven's sin accountants should look at the context. If a guy like Brad Pitt saves himself for marriage he should be allowed to nominate three of his most sinful friends for reprieves on Judgement Day as a tribute to his power over temptation. But if a guy with cystic acne and halitosis saves himself for marriage, then that's just evolution at work.

Deuteronomy then turned to the topic of masturbation. A few nervous giggles were heard but mostly we just stared resolutely at the floor. I was very unsettled because I was hard at it most nights of the week. The first thing he said was that the Bible was silent on masturbation. As far as I was concerned, that was the new good news. He then went on to say that it was important not to let it get out of control and suggested that it be a once-every-two-weeks treat.

"ONCE EVERY TWO WEEKS! I think not, my good man!" is something I wish I had said at the time. I could sense the stirrings of a revolution amongst the assembled wankers and I yearned to lead them in the fight.

I didn't know if his guideline was a scientifically valid rule of thumb or whether he just sucked it out of his own but it struck me as a little strict and made me think that Deuteronomy had forgotten what it was like to be a teenage boy. Following this guideline was his instruction to avoid any lustful thoughts while masturbating. Evidently the Bible says that lustful thoughts are out.

I had not read *1984* at that stage but in retrospect, Christianity began to assume the characteristics of an Orwellian instrument of control. To say that the purely mental experience of lust was wrong was to introduce the notion of thought crimes – a feature of the oppressive dictatorship in Orwell's novel. Did this apply to other negative thoughts like hatred or jealously? Why are my thoughts being monitored by God and equated with sin? Today I can see what a ridiculous concept this was but on that camp it touched a nerve.

I felt dirty and shameful just like on the day my father spoke to me about the sex games when I was ten. Problems with sexuality had led me to Christianity; and sexuality was the reason I eventually lost my faith. Again, adult sexual neurosis - this time in the shape of Deuteronomy - was something I internalised and failed to interrogate. I think that the image of hell in that children's book was so powerful because the corroding guilt I felt about the sex games; and the accompanying belief that I deserved punishment combined to make me susceptible to the notion of a place where sinners went when God came back to judge the world.

I started to obsess about sin. If I masturbated, I felt a devastating guilt and believed that only when I stopped masturbating altogether would I be an acceptable Christian. The most futile exercise was trying to masturbate without fantasising. Although it worked the very first time, that was the last. Imagine me tugging away while desperately trying to concentrate on Maths homework and trying to push away thoughts of Heather Locklear taking off her clothes. It was ultimately unsuccessful because once Miss Locklear got down to her underpants, it was time up for partial differentiation and on with the show.

Chapter III

Mrs Hacking and the missing swearwords

The first significant manifestation of OCD emerged when I was fifteen. It was early evening. I had finished my Biology homework and was packing my books away when an odd thought entered my mind. At first it wasn't accompanied by any emotion. It was simply an inner voice that said, *"What if, by mistake, you have written a swearword or something profane in your homework?"*

Initially, I dismissed it and went to bed, but the thought would not go away. As time wore on, I began to extrapolate and think, "Well, if I did do that, Mrs Hacking would be furious and send me to be beaten." That introduced anxiety into the equation and I started to feel uneasy. I lay in bed for a while and hoped the notion would pass. It didn't. Instead, it became more powerful. After about twenty minutes I was feeling frustrated and thought to myself, "Perhaps I should just read through my homework and set my mind at rest." As I expected, there were no swearwords in the text and I could now get to sleep.

Mrs Hacking was my Biology teacher. She was an excellent teacher but was prone to bouts of rage and irrationality. She was a heavy smoker in her fifties and owned one of the oldest cars in Zimbabwe that I was forced to ride in when she took a friend and me home after bridge club. Bridge club was her idea and not a response to overwhelming demand from the pupils. Members were tricked into signing up for a trial period, after which Mrs Hacking made it almost impossible for them to leave. I was scared of her in class and at bridge club, and was livid with my mother for accepting Mrs Hacking's offer to ferry Adam and me home once a week. Her car had a hole in the passenger side floor through which you could see the road; and on wet days my legs would be sprayed with rainwater. I always found the conversation very strained, especially because my friend was monosyllabic and I felt the need to take up the slack.

At the school, corporal punishment was a feature of the disciplinary practices employed to control miscreant behaviour. At one stage there was some controversy over whether it should be retained and Deuteronomy from the camps, who taught religious instruction at the school, devoted an entire lesson to defending the caning of boys based on the biblical principal of 'spare the rod, spoil the child'. If I had been more intelligent and brave, I would have put up my hand and asked, "Isn't it possible that the rod of discipline is a metaphor, like so much else of the Bible?"

I was terrified of getting beaten. As a result, I was a well-behaved student and no doubt some would say that is proof of corporal punishment's ability to deter bad behaviour. But, in the same way as threatening sinners with hell induces high ratings on the Ten Commandments compliance league tables, my reaction and good behaviour were as a result of fear and not rooted in a moral framework. Corporal punishment is effective, but it is a lazy way to discipline people. Fostering moral behaviour through instruction is much more time consuming and nuanced than inflicting pain.

I think it is possible that a scary teacher and a fear of corporal punishment combined to produce the emergence of OCD that evening in 1991.

Based on what I know now, it is likely that a third factor was involved. Scientific research is tentatively concluding that a genetic predisposition is implicated in the onset and intensification of clinical OCD. A genetic predisposition does not make illness inevitable; it is becoming clear that environmental triggers are required for its emergence.

Fly Fishing For Sharks

Looking back over my life, I can think of quite a few triggers whose influence was insidious and long term, such as guilt and shame linked to religion and sexuality.

With incomplete scientific information causation is difficult to establish at this stage, but I can't help thinking that the anxious little strands of DNA responsible for my illness were activated partly by a combination of religious guilt about my own sexuality; repeatedly failing to repress my own sexuality; and a fear of falling foul of my Biology teacher and ending up bent over a chair while some anachronistic disciplinarian did his level best to create welts on my backside.

I didn't think much about the swearwords incident until the next Biology assignment, when the same thing happened again. Before long it had become a regular pattern and the checking developed into a more and more thorough exercise. It got to the point where I was checking the blank spaces between the words in case I had missed something while reading the actual words. On many occasions, I would close the book after extensive checking and then doubt would begin to eat away at my certainty, so the whole process would begin again. I wasn't totally sure until I got my assignment back from the teacher.

After a couple of months of this time-consuming behaviour, I decided that this thing must come to an end. I resolved that there would be no more checking. Within minutes of packing away the unchecked work my inner voice started to taunt me and, as I resisted, it became more aggressive. It began with statements like:

"Are you sure you didn't write anything disgusting?"
"How do know you didn't?"
"She will definitely send you to be beaten if you did write something."

I started to get agitated and angry that I couldn't convince myself that the work was clear of profanity. Anxiety is an uncomfortable feeling that varies in severity, but it is, in essence, a message from your brain that something is wrong. I was frightened by the anxiety and started to lash out, first with refutation and then with impotent nonchalance:

"Go away, I didn't write anything bad."
"This is just silly."
"I know what I am doing"
"You know, this is not worth it, I don't care if I get beaten."
"Look, just fuck off, I am trying to go to sleep"

My inner voice was aware that, on the contrary, I cared very much about getting beaten and so it upped the ante:

"You motherfucker, you make lots of silly mistakes."
"You have a filthy mind."
"You're a fucking pervert."
"You fucking better check it."

I was now scared and exhausted and the anxiety level was climbing. Like a smoker who can't give up, I climbed out of bed and the checking began.

I didn't think about it at the time, but it is perhaps relevant that the checking for swearwords took place only with Biology homework. Other subjects involved other types of checking – for spelling and accuracy, for example – but that was driven by perfectionism rather than fear of punishment. I wasn't terrified by my other teachers at all, so my homework for them was less emotionally charged.

Other abnormalities began to surface that year. I started becoming obsessed about intruders in my room. This problem emerged after I moved to an outside room that was much bigger and more exposed to potential burglars. Things followed an pattern analogous to the Biology homework. The thought that wouldn't go away was that someone was in my room and would kill me when I was asleep. Perhaps many readers will identify with this concern, as it's natural to be worried about one's safety. Where I probably part company with most people with similar fears, though, is the ritualistic nature of the corresponding compulsions.

It wasn't enough for me to simply close the windows, lock the door and glance around the main room and adjoining bathroom. I would check each wall and the ceilings by dividing them up into segments and scanning each segment individually. The shower would be checked row of tile by row of tile. And all the time I was counting. The eventual number was not important but it was closer to hundred than fifty. On many occasions I would switch off the light and go to bed, but then feel that the checking had not been thorough enough and had to be repeated.

In the second year of this behaviour I developed a new obsession about snakes and, from then on, the room had to be scanned for intruders *and* snakes. The only time that I didn't perform the ritual was when a friend spent the night. The obsession that had been intractable the night before just didn't make an appearance; but it returned as soon as the guest departed.

At about this time something happened that demonstrated what a good Christian I was, if I say so myself. A girl whom I had met implied through friends - as is the way with teenagers - that she liked me. I thought that she was very beautiful but that I didn't stand a chance against other potential suitors. I was still smarting from being called an albino by a girl I had shown interest in. I do have rather translucent eyebrows and below-average stores of melanin but the albino label was inaccurate and unfair. At that time I felt that my appearance was a measure of my worth; and I still think that very little cuts deeper than the knowledge that nobody is turned on by you. I also had a mild case of acne which made me very self conscious and was the subject of many feverish petitions to the Lord for miraculous healing.

If there is a God I think he works for the research and development department at the pharmaceutical company, Hoffman-LaRoche. These were the guys who came up with Roaccutane which cures acne. This stuff is Viagra for teenagers. During treatment you look pretty grim but in the end it works. If only psychiatric drugs were as effective.

After some planning it was arranged for me and this girl to spend time together alone. I was very nervous and unsure of what to say. Sober seduction is not for the faint hearted and I was stumped. I couldn't bring myself to say, "Can I kiss you", so instead I waffled on about rugby - a real favourite with the ladies - and various other soporific topics until she got impatient and came over to where I was sitting and began to kiss me.

As foretold by camp leader Deuteronomy, it wasn't long before my warning light came on. We moved over to lie on the bed and the kissing continued but so did the wretched warning light. Then she said something I'll never forget. Using her naturally seductive tone she whispered, "Any requests?"

I nearly broke into tongues. I was, of course, mightily tempted. Not even in my fantasies had a woman made an offer like that. But the simple fact of the matter is that if I had made a request I would have felt too guilty afterwards. I felt a vain pride at having been so in control of myself that, at the moment when sin beckoned me like a siren, I did not yield. Of course, my secular friends did not see it that way:

they were utterly mystified. Very soon outrage turned to pity
- and pity to mourning for lost opportunities.

Chapter IV

Bleak days with *Bleak House*

I wrote my Cambridge 'O' Level exams at the end of 1992, when I was sixteen. I performed considerably below my potential. It would be self-indulgent to blame it on OCD alone. All the checking for mistakes, tiresome re-reading and swearword fixations certainly blunted my enthusiasm for academic pursuits; but the single biggest factor was good old idleness. We were given very generous study leave and could also stay at home for the entire month and a half over which the exams were written. It was my first experience of freedom because both my parents were working at the time; and I embraced it with glee.

The usual pattern was as follows: up in the morning to attend breakfast, looking as studious as possible; straight to the desk with impressive disregard for distractions, half an hour of study and then as soon as I heard my parents drive off to work, on to my bike and round to my friend's house to kick back and relax.

Between games of pool and catching up on videos I wanted to see, I managed to get enough points to be accepted back to school to begin my 'A' level studies and the final two years of high school. I chose to study Mathematics, Geography and English Literature. I chose Maths because I had taken 'O' level a year early in that subject and somehow got an A grade, which I felt implied some aptitude for the discipline. Or at least that is what I thought. Geography was my favourite subject because I had a fascination with climate and weather. It was also known to be a less rigorous academic pursuit than, say, the natural sciences. English Literature was my mother's idea, although she didn't pressure me to sign up. I was fairly indifferent to literature in general but none of the other subjects on offer seemed very appealing and my mother spoke in awed tones about the delights of Shakespeare, Dickens, Eliot and other people of letters.

It was at the start of 1993, my first 'A' level year, that OCD started its insidious campaign to destroy me. I realise that this sounds dramatic considering the relatively minor complications described thus far but this is all background to the meltdown two years later. The slow battle with schoolwork that began with Biology wore me down so much that when OCD later decided to switch from rubber to metal bullets, my psychological immune system was very weak. Why the military metaphor? Because it was the start of a war that almost killed me.

I had left behind Biology and the swearwords fiasco but now a far more debilitating problem began with English Literature. The first book we had to read was *Bleak House* by Charles Dickens. Until that point in my life, I had done very little reading. I had spent a great deal of time playing sport and if I had a spare couple of hours, I watched TV or visited friends. *Bleak House* is a long book and Dickens uses complicated prose when employing his phenomenal descriptive powers. I felt that I lost track of some of the sentences halfway through. I calculated that I needed to read about fifty pages a week to keep up in class; and, as with all classic procrastinators, I didn't open the book until Sunday of the first week.

As I began to read, there was a growing sense that I hadn't understood or remembered what I had read. I started reading sentences over and over again and yet couldn't suppress the thought that I didn't understand what I had read. By lunchtime, a good four hours later, I was only about ten pages into the book and was feeling exhausted and frustrated. After the meal, I resumed reading but the afternoon was even less productive. I started to get stuck turning the pages. I would struggle to convince myself that I had not turned over two pages instead of one. A ritual developed in which I would have to say the consecutive page numbers out aloud while repeatedly flipping the page over and back again.

"Eighty-three," flip page, "eighty-four." Not convinced, flip page back, "Eighty-three," flip page, "eighty-four." Same doubt comes back, turn over page again, "Eighty-three," flip page, "eighty-four." And so on and so on.

If the page ended in a complete sentence, I would feel the need to check only the page numbers; but if the sentence was broken by the end of the page, I would also get stuck verifying that the text that began on the next page was syntactically connected to the text that ended on the previous one.

And then problems arose with Maths. I think there were two factors that fuelled the OCD in this case. Although I had got an 'A' in 'O' level Maths, the jump to 'A' level was significant. Reasonably hard work was enough at 'O' level but; at 'A' level, diligence had to be combined with aptitude. I started to get wrong answers to many more questions than in the past and felt inadequate at my lack of prowess. Linked to this was a belief I have to this day that if you are not mathematically gifted, you are not a true intellect. My self worth was at stake and the fear of failure and mediocrity ignited the neurotic in me.

It began with me checking that I had copied the examples correctly from the board. I started falling behind because, while the teacher was explaining the principles of a new mathematical concept, I was repeatedly verifying what I had written. Homework became an arduous task because I developed a crippling need to know if my answers were correct before attempting the next problem.

As I write this now, many years later, I am thinking to myself, "Why didn't you just wait to find out after your work was marked?" I do have a vague recollection that I tried to tell myself just to let it go; but the need to know if I was right continued to intensify.

Tests and exams were particularly tense because the fear of making mistakes was magnified. First, there was the repeated re-reading of the question to check that I had understood it - similar to the cycle of repetition with the Dickens novel. Second, there was the checking to see if any information from the question - such as an equation to solve - had to be transferred to the paper I was writing on. Last, there was the double, triple and quadruple checking of each step in the solution once I had come up with the answer. As the checking intensified, so did the anxiety because I was acutely aware that if I spent so much time checking, I wouldn't have time to attempt all the questions. In my final exam I spent about one third of the allotted time checking my work and attempted only two thirds of the questions.

It all became a vicious cycle of decline. Feeding my fear of making mistakes was an entirely rational realisation that I was mathematically average and therefore less likely to solve most of the problems correctly, as I had done with more rudimentary Mathematics in previous years. The checking meant that I wasn't concentrating in class. I wasn't developing my mathematical reasoning abilities because I was doing less and less homework; and I was wasting too much time in tests and exams. In the end I failed my final 'A' level exam. I knew that, even with my limited ability and without OCD, I could have passed with the necessary hard work.

I remember an occasion when my mother came into my room to find me crying. I can't recall what I told her but my tears were as a result of emotional exhaustion from checking my Maths; and frustration at the inertia that stemmed from not being able to move on the next question because I was tormented by a need to know if my previous answer was correct. I had by now lost confidence in my intelligence and was convinced that I made mistakes at every move of my pen. This conviction meant that the vigilant checking seemed necessary, given the obsessive belief in my fallibility.

I've just had a quick chuckle at myself because I looked up 'fallibility' in the dictionary to check the spelling and, in an instant, I flipped into OCD mode. Six double checks later I caught myself and snapped the dictionary shut in disgust. At least with this manifestation of the illness a psychopathological irrationality has become a manageable idiosyncrasy. But whether it is the five and a half pills I take every night or I am actually in control is anyone's guess.

Geography was the least challenging of the three subjects. I had a decent memory so was able to study from the textbook without writing much down. My Geography teacher was an attractive twenty-six-year old woman which meant that the atmosphere in the classroom was permeated with sexual tension - at least among the boys - and this provided a distraction from urges to check my work.

My mother was aware that I was struggling to read the prescribed books for English Literature. She did what most loving mothers do when their child has a problem: she assigned blame to exogenous rather than endogenous factors. My perfectly capable English teacher was denounced at the dinner table for choosing a particular paper from the options available. In 'A' level English Literature, the teacher would choose three papers from about seven that were offered by Cambridge. My mother said that it was ridiculous to expect teenage boys to read *Bleak House* and other tomes; and that my teacher should have chosen another paper. She phoned around and before long I was registered for the Practical Criticism paper which involved minimal reading.

I was taught the remaining two papers at school and on Monday afternoons I received private tuition in Practical Criticism from a wonderful lady, Mrs Davidson. The school was a little affronted by team Alexander and puzzled by this reasonable student who said he couldn't read the prescribed books. I think they thought that I just couldn't be bothered to wade through Dickens and some of his contemporaries. In a fairly benign retaliatory gesture, they made me write the final exams at another school, which unfortunately for me, was a co-ed school. During my Shakespeare paper I was cruelly distracted by a leggy blonde in hot pants sitting across from me which was a difficult adjustment for someone from an all boys' institution. I did poorly in the Shakespeare paper, as a direct result of one part leggy blonde and nine parts insufficient studying. Reading Shakespeare had been as difficult for me as Dickens and I don't think I got to the end of any of the prescribed plays.

I was distressed at my poor academic performance and, with a bruised ego, began to look for something to be good at. In Zimbabwean boys' high schools, the rugby team was often the measure of a school's standing. I was an average rugby player but I was passionate about the game. I was average because I was too afraid of getting hurt to engage properly in the physical confrontation. I was especially tentative when I was up against someone who was bigger and stronger than me. I turned to lifting weights. This not only compensated for my academic decline but also gave me increased confidence on the rugby field. Always supportive, my parents bought me a set of weights that was installed in the courtyard outside my bedroom and I got to work on turning myself into Jean-Claude Van Damme.

Most nights of the week, instead of tearing my hair out over my homework, I would lift weights; and as time went by, I became obsessive about it. Some form of obsession combined with talent is behind most great achievement. But it is a delicate balance: too little, and not much gets done; too much, and you grind to a neurotic halt. My bodybuilding phase was no great achievement but it did combine a modicum of talent and a lot of obsession. Night after night I did bench pressing, squatting and bicep curling and I started to enjoy feeling stronger and more muscular.

The rumour started about six months later, at a swimming gala. I must have made an impression on the spectators because a guy came up to me later and said, "The word on the grapevine is that you are on steroids."

There will always be people who are threatened by success in others and will seek to devalue it in some way. I think I was genetically inclined to develop muscle with the right training and I was quite proud of my physique because I had worked hard for it. The rumour irritated me immensely. Believing that I had taken steroids and had therefore cheated, was a psychological buffer, much like denial, against the realization that they were too lazy to make the sacrifices required by excellence. But who am I to talk? I am always devaluing other people's achievements. The provenance of these thought patterns is my shame about the lack of achievement in my adulthood; and my sense of failure at not having conquered an illness that consists of emotions - albeit very powerful ones - that I didn't consider appropriate for a man. I am starting to accept that I was sick and that it was not my fault that I folded under the pressure but this all takes time.

Fly Fishing For Sharks

It was about this time that I was introduced to the realities of *apartheid*. Nelson Mandela was out of jail but the first democratic elections were still a year away. My school was invited to a rugby tournament in Messina, a town in the Northern Province of South Africa, about twelve kilometres south of the border with Zimbabwe. Teams were invited from all over the province but we were the only Zimbabwean team and hence the only team with black players. We arrived on a dusty evening and parked our bus alongside the school dining hall, outside of which was a crowd of white pupils and a few members of staff who were waiting for us.

The Rugby coach of the host school walked up to us as we disembarked. After a perfunctory greeting, he said: "We don't like kaffirs here. All of the white players will be billeted with parents from the school and the kaffirs will sleep in the dormitory by themselves."

Our coach was outraged. *Apartheid* was supposed to be over and if he had known how our black players would be treated, he would not have attended the tournament. It transpired that there was an unrepealed municipal bylaw in Messina that proscribed blacks and whites from sleeping under the same roof. So the good folk of Eric Louw High School had emptied an entire dormitory for our three black players. They had fifty beds and ten showers all to themselves. Our hosts were not acting out of a reverence for the laws of the land, they were simply using them as a convenient outlet for their bigotry in the last days of white South Africa.

Our coach consulted with us about withdrawing from the tournament but it was decided that this was a splendid opportunity to showcase black athletic talent in rugby, the sport of *apartheid*. One of our black players couldn't make it to the tournament and we all regretted that. He was big, fast, powerful and aggressive but, more importantly, he was an amateur boxer. It would have taken just one racial slur to set him off and there would have been some of Eric Louw's finest writhing on the field, spitting bloody teeth from their shattered jawbones.

I was sent off with a few of my team-mates to stay with a family who owned a game farm. They were very hospitable but the father openly admitted to being a member of the AWB, a right wing organisation for thugs, *apartheid* South Africa's version of the Ku-Klux Klan - and every bit as idiotic - but without the lynching as far as I'm aware. Their English was poor and conversation was dull so I did what I had been taught by my mother, I asked questions:

"What is the population of Messina?"

To which our host replied, "Twelve thousand whites and fifteen thousand animals."

For a brief moment I thought that Messina was a town where people liked to own pets but then I realised that he was referring to blacks. At the time I was, by most measures, a racist. Rhodesia had been a racist society characterised by a watered-down form of *apartheid* and many white Zimbabweans - including myself - had held onto crass prejudices long past independence. But this comment made me ashamed of my racism for the first time. I felt repelled by the way this man felt he could say such a thing while his black domestic worker was nearby.

I was later further disabused of my racist prejudices by two books. I read Nelson Mandela's autobiography and he became my first black role model, as well as eliciting my sympathy for the appalling suffering and degradation that blacks had endured under *apartheid*. Then I read *Guns, Germs and Steel*, a revolutionary book by Jared Diamond. It explains everything you need to know about the divergent development paths that countries and regions have taken throughout history. Professor Diamond shows that the divergence has nothing to do with inherent differences between races and everything to do with geography, climate, flora, fauna and just plain luck.

The tournament itself was a seven-a-side rugby round robin; which meant that there was more emphasis on speed, tactics and ball handling ability than in traditional fifteen-a-side rugby, thus less need for brute force. The players from the Northern Province schools were physically intimidating but not as fast or skilful as our black players. Sevens rugby gives you ample room to run and we had a black player, Owen Chirwa, who was a sprint champion. Try as they might, the South Africans could not catch him and he ran in try after try. It was a pleasure to watch as he shot past opponents whose hysterical parents bellowed futile encouragement in the face of his sheer athletic superiority. Those people, terrified of the political change happening in their country but watching Owen in full stride beating their sons at their own beloved game, found it almost unbearable.

I say 'almost' because the spectators did eventually clap when Owen was given the Player of the Tournament award. The applause was a sign that there was hope for South Africa in the long run. John Maynard Keynes commentated wryly, "in the long run, we are all dead," - here's hoping that South Africans expedite the process of reconciliation voluntarily before it is too late.

South Africa's ANC government has instituted affirmative action and black economic empowerment legislation in attempts to redress the imbalances of *apartheid*. Considering the extent of those imbalances, it is difficult to argue against these corrective measures in theory. In practice, they are creating a society where, once again, race is being used to assign value. I hope that race-based legislation stops at the job market where it has already gone far enough. It would be a terrible irony if post-*apartheid* South Africa became a country where an individual's race determined his or her chances in life. Owen Chirwa won that accolade because he was the most talented player in the tournament.

When he stood up to receive his prize, there was a stony silence from the crowd, broken only by his team-mates' cheers. After about thirty seconds one brave spectator clapped – once. Slowly, the whole crowd began applauding tentatively, then after a while, the clapping became genuine. The long walk to equality had begun for the people of Messina.

On the last night of the tournament, the organisers held a disco in the school hall. We didn't recognise the music – the lyrics were in Afrikaans. The dancing was just as foreign. Teenage couples paired off and engaged in an odd, staccato shuffling, known to the locals as *langarm*. I think the English translation is 'long arm'. This was executed in a strict rectangular pattern that traced the outer perimeter of the dance floor, leaving the centre free for the bemused Zimbabweans. If Patrick Swayze had been forced to teach this type of dance to Jennifer Grey, *Dirty Dancing* would have flopped at the box office. It truly was the least sensual form of physical interaction I have ever seen - but perhaps that was the point.

Even the venerable Deuteronomy would have disapproved of *langarm* because the telltale profile of a fully erect warning light would have been almost impossible to conceal. The *langarming* protocol calls for a safe distance between the bodies of the shuffling couple. The distance would have to be even greater if *langarming* was allowed between same-sex male partners. I think it will be a few generations before Afrikaner religious leaders come to terms with homosexuality. They are still reeling from the shock of discovering that the Bible did not justify *apartheid*. This theological paradigm shift is proving very traumatic for many of them and, as such, setting guidelines for same-sex *langarming* is likely to induce cardiac arrest or - heaven forbid - apostasy.

A few of the Eric Louw boys had baseball caps with swastikas on the front; and one or two had T-shirts with 'Hitler's European tour 1939-45' written across the chest, with a map of Europe showing the sites of the concentration camps. The evening reached a climax when one of our black players asked a white girl to dance. Whether or not there was another municipal bylaw against this sort of thing, I don't know, but some of the Messina boys took exception to it. Tempers flared, threats were made and in the end it was decided that fleeing was the best option. Our team-mate was spirited out of the hall and whisked off to a nearby holiday resort by one of the Zimbabwean parents. Where was the amateur boxer when you needed him?

Chapter V

Crimes of the imagination

1994 was the year when everything changed. It was my final year at high school and my 'A' level results would determine what I could do at university, as well as being the first significant entry on my curriculum vitae. I was made a prefect and head of house, which meant that I was in charge of one quarter of the boys at the school when it came to internal sporting events. I continued to lift weights and OCD continued to play havoc with my academic life.

Two important things happened that year before OCD changed from being an immense source of frustration to a living nightmare. In April, I read an article in *Time* magazine about Wall Street, investment banking and the fascinating world of financial derivatives. Included in the piece was a profile of Goldman Sachs and I remember being amazed by the statistic that it had made more pre-tax profit than the GDP of Zambia. This was before I had studied Economics and learned that most medium-sized, first world cities had more economic significance than Zambia. However, as an ignorant eighteen-year-old I was utterly astounded by this statistic.

What really caught my attention was the fact that the end of year bonuses ranged from one million US dollars for the most junior partner to ten or twenty million for the top dog. Not only was I interested in what I had read about derivatives, I also liked the sound of all that money. This was my testosterone speaking. What I didn't know at the time was that the Goldman Sachs employees earning the big money were such an elite bunch of high achievers that if I was to stand any chance of ever working there, I would need to acquire the following: more testosterone; forty or so IQ points; a quantitative degree (preferably postgraduate) from one of the world's top universities; a better work ethic and, of course, a green card. It did occur to me that in the competitive world of investment banking, I might have to cut down on my obsessive checking if I was to get anything done but I was hoping that whatever it was that was causing my problems would soon find it in its heart to piss off.

The other thing that happened was that I left the Church. I didn't stop believing in God but I felt that if I couldn't control my sexual thoughts, I was not worthy to call myself a Christian. The stumbling block was masturbation. I would make pledges that I would never do it again but within a couple of weeks the need for sexual relief would become too powerful. Corrosive guilt would then set in and I couldn't pray. Christians refer to the tendency to regress to a more sinful life as 'backsliding'. I had been backsliding for about a year and a half: I had tried smoking, started going to nightclubs, discovered swearwords, yoked myself with some unbelievers, dabbled in pornography and stopped going to church.

In March 1994, I had gone to church with some friends and did what any penitent backslider does when he feels he has slid far enough – I recommitted my life to the Lord and thus began the infinitely more difficult process of forwardsliding. Sliding is an inappropriate metaphor because moral regeneration is incremental and arduous with absolutely no smoke breaks. Nonetheless, I was very fired up about this decision and put sin on notice that he and I were parting company because we were in a dysfunctional relationship that was going to force me to blow a significant amount of cash on Judgement Day for a decent defence lawyer.

Within two months, my obsessive quest to conquer sin had come to nothing and I closed my Bible for what I thought was the last time. The burden of guilt had just become too heavy and I was simply not able to avail myself of God's grace, despite the fact that it was reputedly so amazing.

OCD has a very wide range of manifestations and one of them is known as 'scrupulosity'. Essentially, it is an excessively legalistic approach to religion in which the sufferer is tormented by the need to constantly monitor and control his conduct and thoughts to avoid falling out of favour with God. The person never feels secure in God's love and forgiveness, and has an uncertainty about his salvation. For many of my teenage years, I cycled in and out of scrupulosity and eventually gave up on myself as a moral being.

In October that year, I had my last formal class at school followed by study leave for the 'A' level exams which were to take place in November. OCD - although I didn't yet know its name - had taken a heavy toll on my studies and I needed to salvage something from the previous two years in order to gain admission to university. I was motivated by the desire to go to university in Cape Town and the slightly delusional ambition to work on Wall Street.

I was entranced by the natural beauty of Cape Town. An added incentive was that most of my good friends were also planning to go to the University of Cape Town (UCT). We were all excited by a popular myth doing the rounds amongst Zimbabwean teenage boys: in Cape Town there were seven girls for every guy. Fanning the flames of expectation was the popular notion that Capetonian women are famous for their beauty. Capetonian girls *are* spectacular but that statistic was fabrication. (I researched the rumour years later and found that the actual statistic for 1996 was 107 females to every 100 males. In defence of the rumour's progenitor, there was a seven somewhere. Besides, what would a rumour be without a healthy disregard for the facts?)

The 'A' level exam period led to new problems that became unmanageable. I knew that there was a chance that I would fail my exams if I got paralysed by the checking during study and especially during the exam itself. I knew that I had one month to fill in the gaps created by two years of limited academic engagement. I knew that university education was becoming more essential in the job market. And I knew that I wanted to leave Zimbabwe.

My past, my weakness and my desires for the future combined to put me under considerable pressure to make up for the past, conquer my weakness and secure my future. Psychiatric conditions are usually activated during times of extreme stress. Although I had probably had clinical OCD from about sixteen years old, I had managed to hide it from the world. The problem I had with reading was an indicator that something was wrong; but it was a problem that could be avoided by choosing another syllabus and switching to private tuition. Perhaps if I had told my mother about all the other manifestations of the illness, she would have reacted differently.

Everyone experiences stress to a varying degree when writing crucial exams but not everyone loses their mind. Maybe I was weak or maybe I was sick, but I came apart.

It started with a mystical experience on the first night of study leave. I was waiting to fall asleep when I started to experience the odd sensation that my head was sinking down into the bed, while at the same time I became light-headed and cold as if I had low blood sugar levels. In my mind's eye, I was aware of assorted images of human activity that became progressively more frenzied. After a couple of minutes of this I thought I should sit up, turn on the light and get some fresh air.

The light switch was on the wall about a metre above my bed. I sat up in the dark and tried to switch it on. I became a little anxious when, after pushing the switch with my finger, it didn't budge. I tried again and again until eventually I started hitting it with the palm of my hand in a flat panic. It was as if my hand was a holographic projection with no substance. I then turned my head and saw myself lying on the pillow. I blacked out. The next thing I remember I was sitting on the edge of the bed with my feet on the floor and the light on. I felt very uneasy.

I think that, in a way, even on a symbolic level, some part of me left that night as if it had seen what was coming and decided that it could not cope.

A few days later, I had to pick up my brother from school because my mother was at a business meeting. As with most junior school parking lots, it was reasonably chaotic at the day's end, with cars jostling for position and excited children running to greet their parents. About twenty minutes after I returned home I was back at my desk and, out of the blue, a very disturbing and emotionally loaded thought originated somewhere in my brain. I was seized by the idea that I had run over and killed a child with my car in the bustling school parking lot. The anxiety associated with this thought was so powerful that I had to rush to the toilet and vomit. It was frightening and confusing because part of me did not remember anything remotely like the catastrophe that was playing out in my mind.

Some years later I read an academic paper on OCD which postulated that in some types of the illness, the brain fails to adequately distinguish between something imagined and something that actually took place. This has not been proven

46

but it makes a lot of sense to me as I look back over the years; and at that first incident in 1994 in particular. The part of the brain that was causing my anxiety is much older in evolutionary terms than other parts of the brain. It is made up of the essential structures that regulate our 'fight or flight' response to danger and hence was crucial to the survival of early humans who lived in the wild. Of course, it still serves us well in today's world with all its threats. The 'fight or flight' response allows us to perform abnormal acts of aggression or retreat in a way that would not be possible without the threat of danger.

Physiological changes moderated by the brain - including a surge of adrenalin - prepare the body for extremes of exertion. Because this mechanism evolved earlier in man's developmental history than other parts of the brain, it causes an instinctive response that is not initially dependent on cognitive contributions from these other parts, such as the frontal lobes, which are responsible for our intellectual superiority over other creatures. The 'fight or flight' response is not only independent of the newer parts of the brain for activation but is also almost impossible to override in the face of a real threat. We have all been told at some time in our lives that if we find ourselves in a certain situation – be it an earthquake, shark tank, snake pit, riot or hijacked plane – the last thing to do is panic. Alas, for most of us, that is the first thing we do and people with anxiety disorders like OCD are some of the best panickers of all.

Anxious hunter-gatherers were more likely to survive and anxiety is an adaptive emotion in certain situations. OCD is at base a maladaptive response to uncertainty and the fact that we are mortal beings whose environment is sometimes hostile to life. However, it is linked to the 'fight or flight' response which is one of the reasons that humans are still here, rather than extinct. In their attempts to insulate themselves from the threats of an unpredictable world, some

OCD sufferers destroy their lives. The attempt to insulate oneself is simply a response to a much higher level of perceived danger as a result of a faulty 'fight or flight' panic mechanism that is in overdrive. In a serious clinical case of OCD, the sufferer is simply obeying a brain that is continually telling him that he should panic. When no visual threat is observed, the imagination fills in the gaps – and the imagination has the power to create as well as destroy.

If the hypothesis in the paper is correct - and in my case it does seem to make sense then it is possible that the surge of anxiety and subsequent vomiting was because some part of my brain had reacted to the thought about killing the child as if it had actually happened. I was engaging the rest of my brain with everything I had in an attempt to refute the thought and ease the anxiety. Almost all the compulsive behaviour witnessed in OCD is an attempt to lessen anxiety. If I had experienced that thought with no anxiety I probably would have forgotten about it relatively quickly. But a part of my brain that I was not programmed to ignore was screaming fight or flight. How do you run from a thought that will not go away? Or how do you fight it? If I had sprinted up the street as if fleeing from a rabid dog, the thought would have come along for the ride; and if I had punched my head in aggression, I would have had an aching skull as well as acute anxiety.

There seemed to be only one solution. I had to get into the car, drive back to the school and scour the parking lot for evidence of culpable homicide.

The anxiety was exacerbated by the worst-case scenario extrapolations that my mind spun out from the initial thought. I imagined being arrested and charged with killing a child, followed by an extended trial with hysterical parents screaming invective as I was led out from the holding cells into the courtroom.

Leading on from those images, I felt tortured by the thought of being sentenced to a lengthy prison term in one of Harare's appalling prisons. Zimbabwe's population was ninety-nine percent black and so most of the prisoners were also black: I felt that I would be the subject of racial attacks. I was besieged by thoughts of being raped repeatedly. These thoughts raised the spectre of contracting AIDS which at that time was a death sentence.

The fear of being trapped in Zimbabwe and not going to UCT only increased the need to be sure I hadn't killed someone. If I didn't return to the school to check the parking lot, I could see no end to the thoughts and the anxiety; not to mention the fact that I was already behind in my revision and the little I had done was marred by increased obsessive checking that I can only attribute to the desperate need to pass.

I drove back to the school to find that, of course, there was not a hint of the aftermath of a tragic accident. The interplay of the anxiety with the original persistent thought and accompanying extrapolations transformed what were admittedly abnormal cognitive phenomena into full-blown obsessions. Such was the discomfort that a compulsive urge to neutralize that feeling led me back to the school. At the time I did not see any other way out. I did not know that this sickness had a name and I felt totally out of control. The academic troubles had been frustrating but this was horrible.

I went to bed that night - after checking for intruders and snakes - hoping that what had come that day would not visit me again.

In order to counter the checking involved in studying, I began to read material onto cassette tapes that I then listened to again and again, hoping to absorb the knowledge. In this way I managed to lessen the impact of the re-reading compulsions but found it hard to concentrate on the material because my anxiety levels were high. This strategy was partially successful in Geography and English; but Maths was about mastering concepts and doing examples. There was just not enough time to repair the damage.

Although I didn't do much driving at that time, the 'incident' at the school was the beginning of a number of obsessions associated with driving. Pedestrians and cyclists were the focus of the growing neurosis. Did I hit that cyclist or knock his pedal and cause him to swerve off the road into a tree? Did he die from his injuries? Did I run over that pedestrian? Did I reverse over a small child that I couldn't see in my rear view mirror as I was pulling out of a parking space? I was continually looking in my rear view mirror to check that the cyclist, pedestrian or child wasn't lying lifeless and bloody on the road.

OCD had a new obsession for every neutralising strategy that I resorted to. For example, it would ask,

"While you were checking for dead people in the rear view mirror, did you kill someone who you hadn't seen in front of you?"

This increased the compulsive response so that before I checked the rear view mirror, I had to scan the road ahead a few times to check for potential victims. On almost all occasions, I would not be content with just one glance in the rear view mirror. I was however, often able to limit the number of glances to three or four before I felt safe. But if OCD was firmly in the driver's seat, I was unable to trust the sensory data being processed in my brain - regardless of the number of rear view mirror confirmations - that I hadn't killed anyone.

In all these instances, the 'victim' was either out of sight or I had turned into another road before I had stopped checking. The doubt and anxiety would grow; the fear of the consequences of culpable homicide would mount and I would stop the car, turn around and retrace my journey to assure myself that I had not killed anyone. Often I would lose track of the cyclist which would compel me to scour the neighbourhood in order to see that he was cycling along happily.

If the obsession hit me soon after I had driven past the potential victim, I could usually lessen the anxiety by checking in the rear view mirror. But if the obsession struck later the next day or at any time when it was too late or simply impossible to get back into the car, my only option was to try and reconstruct the journey in my mind from start to finish; and mentally retrace the route again and again until I was comfortable that nothing had happened. Sometimes the retracing would take minutes, sometimes hours. In extreme circumstances it could take months of intermittent rumination before the calm returned.

This reconstruction was a compulsion in the same way as checking in the rear view mirror or scanning my homework for swearwords - the only difference being that it would not have been visible to an observer. This type of OCD is known as Pure-O.

I drove myself to my Maths exam but I was running late, which meant that I drove faster than I was comfortable with. Speeding exacerbates my OCD: perhaps because of a combination of guilt, a reduced checking timeframe and the knowledge that any accident would be more severe as a result the physics of speed. I knew that speeding would also be an aggravating factor in the eyes of the judge when the case came to trial.

On the way to the exam, I passed a cyclist on a convex section of the road and by the time I looked in my rear view mirror he was almost out of sight. Ordinarily, I would have driven back to be absolutely certain that he was unharmed, but there wasn't time.

That Maths exam was brutal. I couldn't concentrate because I was thinking about the cyclist and this added anxiety compounded the obsessive checking of my work. The entire three-hour paper was saturated with neurosis. Unsurprisingly, I failed. Well, I actually got a subsidiary pass which is not quite a failure; but it is not much of an achievement either. The symbol on the results sheet for a subsidiary pass is 'O'. It might as well have stood for Obsessive.

Most mornings in the shower I would now vomit from anxiety because I sensed that I was losing touch with reality and it terrified me. I was fighting with my sister about her boyfriend because I was irrationally angry about their relationship and the possibility that it might become sexual. He was a fantastic guy called Alex and we had started to become good friends leading up to the relationship. But something about my sister's path to womanhood made me irrational and protective; although, because of my immature emotional processes, it manifested itself as just plain nastiness. I was increasingly alienated from my parents because of my approach to my sister's partner; and it all came to a head when I refused to lend him some very helpful study material that I had been given by a friend.

We both did English Literature and he would have benefited from access to this material. On discovering that I had hidden the material in my cupboard, my mother - who by this stage had had enough of my behaviour - threw her coffee at me and said that I was "fucking warped". She was right. I was. I have forgiven her for that comment because I realise how frustrated she must have been with me. The distressing fact of the matter is that she had hit the nail on the head. But still I didn't tell anyone what was happening to me.

Towards the middle of November, another obsessive theme emerged as the illness tightened its grip. At the time, Zimbabwe was coming to terms with the AIDS pandemic and hospital beds were starting to fill with the sick and dying. I was not aware that there was effective medication for the virus and - for someone who was petrified of death - even the mention of the acronym made me shudder. I knew that it was a sexually transmitted disease and that the only other means of transmission were sharing infected needles or receiving a transfusion of contaminated blood. I was not sexually active, I was not an intravenous drug user and I had never received a blood transfusion. Logically, I was safe.

One morning I was putting a video cassette back into its plastic box and I cut my finger very slightly on one of the edges. There was a miniscule amount of blood but the cut did not warrant a plaster. A couple of minutes later an extremely bizarre and morbid thought took hold of me.

"There might have been contaminated blood on the plastic box, and because you cut yourself, you might have AIDS."

I immediately refuted the notion as ridiculous but the thought persisted. It persisted in spite of a continuous flow of logical reasons why it was not possible for me to be HIV positive.

Persistent thoughts are potent tools of psychiatric illnesses. The longer OCD can keep a distressing thought in your mind, the more damage it can do because the longer a person is focussed on that thought, the worse the anxiety will become; and the worse the anxiety becomes, the more frenzied the attempts to counter the psychological pain.

Imagine for a minute that you are in a committed relationship with someone and there is absolutely no evidence to suggest that your partner is being unfaithful to you. One day the thought pops into your head that your partner is starting to cheat on you. Rationally, you know it to be highly unlikely and you rebut the thought in disgust. But it continues to bother you throughout the day and into the evening. It bothers you not because it might be true but simply because you can't stop thinking about it. After a couple of days or weeks, the thought will spawn one of two responses. These responses might be expedited by the experience of intermittent episodes of lurid mental images of your partner making love to someone else – images that might intensify while the two of you are making love.

The first and most destructive response to your obsession - for that is what is has become - is to give the notion some credibility and let it influence your behaviour towards your partner. The second response is to try to end your ordeal by simply asking your partner for reassurance that your thoughts are wrong. This might help if the thought goes away.

But if it persists and the images taunt you further, you might become stuck in a cycle of continually asking for reassurance from your partner. If this does not help, you might start checking his or her e-mails and cell phone just to make sure.

I have deliberately used the emotionally charged subject of infidelity to enable you to enter the mind of someone who is not in control of his thoughts. Infidelity, or even the suspicion of infidelity, has ruined lives since antiquity and is an area of human behaviour that is replete with obsessive lust and compulsive urges. Have you ever been compelled by lust to do something that could ruin your life and the lives of those close to you? Are you driven by a need to sleep with someone other than your partner just to know the orgasmic delights of forbidden fruit? Does the thought of someone having sex with the love of your life make you sick to your core? The content of the obsessions and the motives for the compulsions are different in OCD; but the ruined lives, psychological torture and emotional intensity are all there.

The AIDS obsession, like the killing-a-child obsession before it, eventually drove me back to the scene of the 'incident'. I took the plastic box outside into the full sunlight and searched for blood. The box was clean - at least to the naked eye - and I had some temporary relief. I actually thought that there was a little plausibility in my obsession. If there had been blood on the box and if my cut had been subcutaneous, there would have been - in my mind - a minute chance that the virus could enter my bloodstream. The blood would need to be fresh and contaminated but I consoled myself afterwards that I was not being utterly ridiculous in checking the box.

The foundation of a good prognosis for a neurotic patient is that he recognises that his behaviour is irrational and wants to stop. The difficulty with psychotic patients is that they generally lack insight into their conditions and are thus less in touch with reality. The fact that I thought that checking the box was even nominally rational was, in hindsight, an indication of the increasing severity of my illness.

Within days the obsession had spread to a dread of any contact between my skin and another surface. Because our hands are the parts of the body that most often touch other things, the obsessive focus honed in on my hands. The level of irrationality increased such that I was convinced that if contaminated blood came into contact with my skin, it would seep through and enter my bloodstream. AIDS symbolised death. And death was once again the end result of the extrapolation projected from the original obsession.

After I had touched something like a door handle, the anxiety would spike and I would scrutinise every inch of my inner hand for signs of blood. The scrutiny would be immediate if no-one else was present; delayed if I had company; and clandestine if I thought I could get away with it. Our palms - or at least my palms - have a blotchy pinkish-red colouration that is not a great source of solace when you are checking for blood. As was the case when driving, I did not trust my own eyesight and I began to supplement the visual checking with compulsive hand washing – a feature of OCD that many people are familiar with.

At times I was under the illusion that I was one step ahead of OCD and so began to check objects before I touched them to forestall the anticipated anxiety. As a result, before the extensive hand washing could begin, the taps, the soap and the towel had to be checked for blood because I believed nothing was safe.

I was one step ahead alright but only on the path to paranoia. Because within two months, I started to believe that someone was stalking me with a syringe full of contaminated blood that he squirted onto things that I was likely to touch. I began checking my cutlery for blood before eating a meal, a habit that persisted for many years.

It was all becoming tiresome and I decided that I was going to avoid dealing with my problems by using the one method that has stood the test of time – getting drunk. This was a huge decision for me because at the tender age of eleven and a half I had made a vow with my closest friend that we would never drink. There had been alcoholism in his extended family and - after we had witnessed a family friend get out of hand one evening - we took the decision to protect ourselves from the perils of liquor by declaring our own little Prohibition.

For most of my teenage years this dovetailed nicely with my religious convictions and I got quite a kick out of refusing any offers of tainted beverages. I felt superior. I looked upon drinkers - especially the vomiting adolescent experimenter who didn't know his limit - as a degenerate breed of humans who had no regard for their health or dignity. My distaste was heightened by careful study of the Book of Proverbs which was pretty clear that excessive drinking was not on or, at least, was a stumbling block to wisdom. The author of this finger-wagging bit of the Bible turned out to be Solomon, King of Israel, who was wise enough to keep a bevy of concubines on call. I suppose if you are having as much sex as Solomon the Wise, you probably don't need to drink.

A friend of mine who had no intention of passing his exams because he didn't want to go to university, volunteered to have a party at his house partly motivated, no doubt, by the prospect of my stated intention of getting drunk for the first time. He lived nearby and so I walked to the party. I had an intuitive sense that drunk driving would lead to more bizarre obsessions, particularly if my mind was allowed to fill in the blanks left by memory loss which I understood to be a possible side effect of heavy drinking. It was also illegal and, although my moral compass was beginning to change direction without the magnetic pull of religion, I was still a law-abiding fellow at heart.

There were no girls and no parents at the party and the evening developed into an orgy of Pilsner, peach Schnapps and pirated pornography – a genre that I had hitherto rejected as a base and tasteless art form. I still think it's base and tasteless but that does not detract from its entertainment value. I consider adult pornography to be a useful tool and a tribute to libertarianism's triumph over the sort of people who think that privacy is a suspect notion.

I staggered back home, swigging from a bottle of beer that I had brought along for company. My mother was awake and I made my best effort to appear sober when she greeted me at the end of the corridor. What I should have said was, "Mom, something terrible is happening to me and I am so scared – please help me." Instead, I engaged her in conversation as if she was an old colleague I had bumped into on a brisk morning walk. Everything I said was louder than I had intended and delivered with an exaggerated politeness and poorly executed alacrity in an attempt to wrap up the conversation as quickly as possible to avoid any probing questions. The offending bottle had been hidden in the garden as a precaution.

"Greetings mother, what a surprise. Have you had a good evening?"
"Andrew, you are very late."
"Better late than never, dear maternal unit."
"Have you been drinking?"
"I had a beer or two with Cawood and the boys."
"But you don't drink."
"Strictly speaking, I don't, but in the last little while, I have been wondering what....oops, bugger it...I completely forgot about these bloody steps."
"Are you drunk?"
"Difficult to say for sure, but I feel I must go to bed as immediately as possible. Lovely chatting to you, mom, see you at breakfast."
"Good night darling....sleep tight."

It is hard to accurately convey the experience of your first serious hangover. Effectively, you have poisoned yourself and your body is in shock. Vomiting, nausea, spectacular headaches – the experience will be familiar to many readers.

Fly Fishing For Sharks

It was such a traumatic experience for me that I went through the entire grief cycle that usually accompanies your impending death or the loss of a loved one. On the third or fourth vomiting spree, I spewed up what looked like blood and that is when an untimely death, I dramatically concluded, became something I could not rule out entirely.

First up in the grief cycle was the denial. I thought that it was impossible that alcohol alone could be responsible for my symptoms and I was convinced for a while that I had come down with some strange tropical ailment. When my mother came to check on me, I groaned plaintively that I had been stricken with malaria. I knew nothing about malaria but it seemed like a bad thing to have and it would elicit more sympathy than a hangover.

Next was the bargaining stage. I made firm resolutions to resurrect my vow to my friend and hoped that these good intentions would speed my recovery. But there was no respite. Hot on the heels of the bargaining came the depression, not clinical Depression but self-pity, followed by self-recrimination as I segued into the anger stage of the cycle. I chastised myself for breaking the vow, for my lack of self-discipline and for not drinking water before I went to bed as instructed.

It was well into the afternoon before I moved from anger to the last stage of the grief cycle – acceptance. I reluctantly had to admit to myself that I had drunk too much, and that I must take full responsibility for the morning of anguish. I did experience that exquisite sense of relief that accompanies the first realisation that your hangover is over. It is a feeling that almost makes binge drinking worthwhile.

Chapter VI

Eighteen holes of therapy

I am going to put 1994 on hold here and attempt, instead, to analyse my OCD so far. The analysis is informed mainly by a flamboyant Serbian psychiatrist whom I saw some years later for about six months.

An old paradigm in psychiatry holds that if, through extensive analysis of his past, a patient can gain insight into the source of his neurosis, he would be provided with some relief from his symptoms. This was known - and probably still is - as the talking cure. Obviously, my past influenced the specific manifestations of OCD that I experienced but knowing the dynamics of that interaction did not give me any relief from symptoms. In fact, they only intensified under stress as soon as I stopped seeing the Serbian fellow.

OCD is a poorly understood mental illness that appears to be influenced by genetic, neurochemical and neurophysiological abnormalities which, once activated, can lead to a chronic condition that no amount of therapy can entirely reverse for similar reasons that couch time would be ineffective against diarrhoea. Therapy has its place in mild cases and can help in managing the disorder but its utility is limited.

OCD ranges in severity from slightly annoying and mildly time-consuming to almost total disability. I know from reading books and talking to other sufferers that I had a severe form of the disorder and I will feel vindicated if, one day, science shows me that I had no reason to feel ashamed of myself for not overcoming the illness; in the same way that people who develop other illnesses unrelated to their lifestyle choices, are not seen as complicit in their misfortune.

The man I mentioned at the beginning of this book who said that other people had worse problems than me but still soldiered on, was implying that if I was more of a man and a stronger person, then I would be able to pull myself together and get on with life. As I said, he was right. Hundreds of millions of people are worse off than I am. But how is that relevant to my experience of mental illness? When I think of other people who are worse off than me but are coping better, I simply feel guilty that I am not empowered by the knowledge of my comparatively good fortune to take charge of my life.

Having said all this, I think it's worth taking a moment to review some of the psychodynamic theories that I have developed as well as the original hypothesis put forward by the Serbian. You may have seen this coming but the Serbian believed that the accumulated guilt associated with my childhood sexual experimentation had played a crucial role in the development of OCD. He summed up my self-image thus: "I am a bad boy who makes bad mistakes that have bad consequences."

To hear him rant about how many adults are confused and hypocritical about sexuality was very reassuring; and his summaries of the academic literature about the widespread incidence of childhood sexual exploration and its role in healthy development were equally comforting. He was an intense and passionate individual who had fought in the Balkans war. If nothing else, our sessions were entertaining. By the time I walked into his office in August 2000, I was a smoker and the two of us puffed away until the air in his office was about as potent as what we were happily inhaling into our lungs. In what was probably a breach of accepted psychiatric protocol, we even played a few rounds of golf together.

When I told him about what we had been taught about masturbation and lustful thoughts at those camps, he erupted into a paroxysm of rage and invective directed against the deleterious effects of organised religion on human sexuality. It was all very liberating. He was also deeply distrustful of the global pharmaceutical industry. As a result, I spent six months on almost no medication and developed a slight tranquiliser habit. However, I wasn't working and probably drove only twice a week which meant that I was under so little stress that I managed to muddle through that period without coming apart.

I have jumped the gun slightly by introducing the Serbian theory because when I started seeing him, five years had passed since I'd been diagnosed with OCD. But I have done so in order to give you a basis for comparison with any theories you might develop as you read this book.

My theory is that once I abandoned religion, there arose in me an unacknowledged awareness that if I died, I would no longer be protected from hell. I had heard about the unforgivable sin against the Holy Spirit and I suspected that I might be guilty of it by virtue of my apostasy. Apostasy is perhaps a melodramatic noun in this case. I stopped going to church because I was losing the battle with sin, not because I thought that a belief in God was untenable. I did not stop believing in God; I felt that he had stopped believing in me. I wonder how many other Christians around the world think that a suppression of their sexuality is mandated by their faith. I am thinking particularly of gay and lesbian people who might be tortured by the notion that they are an abomination to God. The only abominable thing about it is that God is petty and insecure enough to get his knickers in a knot about what loving couples do in the privacy of their own home. "God, why don't you spend a few Sunday afternoons making genocide a thing of the past and stop wasting time defining the gender parameters of love – it really is *so* Old Testament."

The OCD that began with the Biology homework had been frustrating but what emerged during my final exams was terrifying and linked with the fear of death. There was a six-month lag between leaving the church and the emergence of this latter type of OCD. Proposing a causal link is certainly inviting refutation but I think I am onto something. The early OCD was linked to a fear of the consequences of making mistakes - particularly corporal punishment - which might have been my reaction to how bad I felt about the childhood sex play (my biggest mistake to date) whose attendant guilt could have bred an obsessive fear of feeling so dirty again. The sudden arrival of death as a theme in the illness meant that the Obsessive-Compulsive cycle was fuelled by a stronger fear and hence became more crippling.

The fear of death had surfaced in a milder form when I began to check my room for intruders and snakes. The fear of contamination with AIDS-carrying blood does relate to death but also has strong undercurrents of sexual guilt. It does seem plausible that my childhood experience of guilt combined with a crisis of faith centred on masturbation and lustful thoughts to produce a person who saw himself as a damned soul who had to avoid death at all costs.

These psychological factors influenced the specific manifestations of my OCD; while the stress of final exams must have triggered the full expression of the genetic predisposition. This could have activated other neurological abnormalities responsible for the new symptoms. Given the earlier signs of OCD, this process must have begun a few years previously.

By Christmas 1994, I was very ill.

The exam period finally came to an end and shortly afterwards the Alexander family went on holiday to Cape Town. With the stress of exams removed, I found that I could cope slightly better with life. The morning vomiting became less frequent as the anxiety dropped below its peak; and I kept telling myself that everything would be fine once I had been accepted by UCT. I think some measure of optimism and denial is crucial when dealing with any crisis. How I thought I was going to get a degree in finance with my obsessive checking and mathematical mediocrity, is a mystery to me. For that matter, how was I going to drive to work if I thought that I was killing cyclists en route and causing accidents? I suppose I was young and scared and the only thing that kept me going was a belief that my troubles were temporary.

I was desperate to leave Zimbabwe and excited at the thought of studying in Cape Town. Thanks to Roaccutane, I was cured of acne and felt ready to capitalise on the mythical seven-girls-to-one-boy ratio. This projection of success with girls was a graphically implausible extrapolation from my dismal track record in Harare. It was predicated on the naïve conception that the only thing that had been holding women at bay was the proliferation of zits on my face. It turned out that there was a lot more to sex appeal than clear skin and that, for each beautiful Capetonian woman, there was an extremely handsome fellow with a hometown advantage and considerably more disposable income. To add insult to injury, Zimbabwean female students on arrival in Cape Town generally concluded that their male counterparts compared poorly to the South African talent pool.

About two weeks into the holiday, a bizarre obsession emerged. It became the catalyst for my first breakdown early in 1995. I was walking along a beach on my own in the late afternoon sun. It was windy and the periodic thud of the breaking waves was the only sound I heard. The beach was about eight kilometres long and over a kilometre wide in places; and it became progressively more deserted as I walked south, away from the holiday resort at the northern end where we were staying. By the time the obsession made an appearance, there was no-one within five hundred metres of me. As in my other obsessions, the thought was accompanied by strong anxiety that combined with the intractability of its intrusion into my conscious mind to produce enough distress to compel a response. However, this thought was so bizarre that I was able to delay the compulsive reaction longer than usual. I was so taken aback at the irrationality of the thought that before I responded to it, I remember saying to myself, "Andrew, if you look over your shoulder to combat this thought, you are really in trouble because this will be the start of a meltdown."

The obsession was that I had stepped on a baby and killed it. Initially, I carried on walking but my pace slowed as I fought the terrible images in my head. I came to a halt, my heartbeat audible above the sound of the waves. I stared rigidly ahead as the terror grew, and the desire to check began to overwhelm me.

After fighting the urge to look back over my shoulder for as long as I could, I succumbed to the panic and turned my head to scan the beach behind me for evidence of the image that I could not dismiss from my mind. All I saw were footprints being slowly filled in by a continuous film of sand that was gliding over the beach in the wind.

The consequential extrapolations that led to the backward glance were similar to those involved in driving: prison, rape, AIDS and death. In addition, there was the horror and guilt at the thought that I might have killed a defenceless child.

Why didn't I summon up everything I had and refuse to look back? If I had, maybe I would have been able to turn the tide of the illness and reduce the other compulsions as well. The problem was - and still is - that OCD sufferers want absolute certainty that the thing they fear has not happened. Some part of my brain knew that it was unlikely that I had stepped on a baby and killed it without knowing; but another part was acting as if it had happened. Without that guarantee that nothing had happened, I could not rule out the possibility of experiencing the horrors that awaited me in prison if I was found guilty of such a careless murder.

For me to not look back over my shoulder was the equivalent of saying that I did not fear prison, rape and death. However hard I tried to come to terms with those outcomes, I could never think of them as anything but unacceptable and to be avoided at all costs, even if it meant losing my mind and becoming a prisoner of fear. As I said earlier, maybe I was weak or maybe I was ill but when push came to shove, I had to look over my shoulder because I felt my life depended on it.

On a couple of occasions that holiday I resolved not to respond to my obsessions; but within hours I could not bear the anxiety anymore and resumed the compulsions. The baby-killing obsession meant that everywhere I walked I glanced over my shoulder to see if there was a body. It didn't seem to matter whether I was in a crowded shopping mall or on a deserted beach. It was irrelevant that in a crowded shopping mall or on a busy pavement, a baby lying on the ground would cause a commotion. These aspects of reality were immaterial to me and I had to be vigilant. Opening doors also became an issue because I might have squashed a baby against the wall when I entered a room. I would check my hands for blood that might have been on the doorknob and then glance behind the door to check that there was no baby.

I did drive a little during that holiday but only if other people were in the car. I felt safe if this was the case because they would act as my witnesses at the trial if something happened. I trusted their senses but not mine. In years to come, this would change but - for the first year or so - a passenger was a great blessing to me. My brother, whom I love dearly, was only twelve when I was diagnosed and there was a very touching moment when I had to take him across town to a friend's house. We had told him a bit about the illness but, because we didn't want to scare him, he was given a slightly watered down version of the symptoms. Nonetheless, he was bound to pick up other details and this became clear to me on that day when I offered him the front seat of the car but he declined.

"I'll sit in the back and look out the window in case you need me to tell you that nothing happened."

"Thanks, Rory, I really appreciate that."

It was a loving gesture from a kid who did not know how else to help. Little things like that help to put families back together again after mental illness has shattered their lives and strained relationships to breaking point. A supportive family is a vital adjunct to medication.

Chapter VII

Free will and chocolate mousse

You might have noticed that when talking about my obsessions I use terms such as 'might have', 'what if' or 'possibly' before describing an imagined scenario. I once described OCD as 'the tyranny of what ifs' and I still think that statement sums up the basic dynamic of the illness. In almost all cases, the 'what if' scenario is highly implausible and it would be useful to discover what it is about the OCD sufferer's brain that is so different that the overwhelming implausibility of the feared event does not seem to attenuate the disproportionate emotional response.

I believe that the authors of the paper I cited earlier were on to something when they suggested that certain types of OCD result from a cognitive processing malfunction in which the brain fails to adequately distinguish between a mental image and a visual perception. That would account for the activation of the 'flight or fight' mechanism which is well understood. I hope that science will soon uncover the neurological dynamics of the hypothesised cognitive processing malfunction and find more successful interventions for treatment-resistant patients.

Some OCD patients - including me - have what is known as 'treatment-resistant OCD'. This refers to an OCD symptom profile that is unresponsive to any of the Selective Serotonin Reuptake Inhibiters (SSRIs), a class of psychiatric drugs that constitute the opening salvo of any pharmacological assault on the illness. They are a subgroup of anti-depressants of which Prozac is probably the most well-known example. As far as I know, there are no drugs specifically designed for OCD. Part of the reason for this is that the physiopathology and biochemistry of the illness are so poorly understood. If the pharmaceutical industry doesn't know exactly what is wrong, it should come as no surprise that their drugs have a limited efficacy in relieving symptoms.

Prozac is indicated for Major Depression, Bulimia Nervosa and OCD, amongst other conditions. Is this vast range of psychopathology all because of the abnormally high re-uptake of serotonin in the patients' synaptic clefts? Surely the brain, which has about a hundred billion neurons, is not an organ for which such reductionism is even heuristically appropriate? As Demi Moore said to Tom Cruise in *A Few Good Men* when he was trying to oversimplify the case they were working on, "You're gonna have to go deeper than that." I'm sure Shakespeare had something far more eloquent and perspicacious to say to the pharmaceutical industry than Ms Moore did to Mr Scientology; but I probably got stuck turning the pages of one of his plays and discarded the book in frustration before I got to it. Hollywood screenplays served me poorly in my English Literature exam but I simply can't resist quoting them.

It turns out to be much more complicated than serotonin in the synapses. According to Robert M. Sapolsky in *Why Zebras Don't Get Ulcers,* the jury is still out on whether it is too little or too much serotonin that is implicated in Depression. In addition, there can be up to fourteen types of serotonin receptors at the end of a single neuron. And even when anti-depressants are effective - and they are often anything but - it can be up to six weeks before the symptoms begin to moderate. This is because the altered levels of serotonin in the synaptic clefts are only the beginning of a process that effects changes further along the neuronal pathway. This chain reaction is only marginally understood but its mechanisms must surely hold a few grooves in the key to unlocking the mystery of Depression and OCD. Why do some patients respond but not others? One of the risks associated with Depression is suicide. People are killing themselves as you read this and will continue to do so until we can answer this question.

The frustration that mentally ill people feel with their partial remissions, residual symptoms and - in some cases - complete lack of progress, must be felt by many patients right along the medical spectrum whose illnesses are resistant to medical advances. I can only speak for psychiatry when I say that doctors should be more forthright about how little they know about the mind and therefore how difficult it is to treat a patient with a serious mental illness. Such openness might come as a shock to the sufferer but at least it would be honest and would remove the likelihood of the sufferer clinging to a leaking lifeboat of false hope. I know, because mine sank.

In his book *The Madness of Adam and Eve*, David Horrobin said the most advanced anti-psychotic drugs are capable of treating only about 20 per cent of the symptoms of Schizophrenia. What's more, that 20 per cent gain is partially lost when the side effects of the drugs are factored into a quality of life consideration. When I read about the bland existence that characterises the lives of so many medicated schizophrenics and other psychiatric patients, a frustrated despondency erodes my confidence that advances in science will lead to the discovery of cures.

My fourth psychiatrist once told me that I was in remission - according to the textbook definition of the term. Admittedly, by the time I saw him I could drive to my appointment without thinking that I had killed someone on the way; and when I sat down in his office I didn't check the chair for blood. However, he and his predecessors had made very little headway in addressing the OCD that almost wiped out my academic life and was still sabotaging my ability to hold down even the most menial job.

Fly Fishing For Sharks

A major improvement in my symptom profile (the obsessions about contaminated blood and killing people while driving) was achieved with the addition of anti-psychotic medication - traditionally used for Schizophrenia - to my prescription list. By the late 1990s, atypical anti-psychotics were being used in addition to the SSRIs for the management of treatment-resistant OCD. I first learnt of the correct dosages for this strategy from a friend in the United Kingdom and not from my psychiatrists. It was late 2002 and I had experienced two major relapses since the knowledge of how to manage treatment-resistant OCD had come to light. This friend was a doctoral student in immunology and could access academic journals online from her laboratory. I had asked her to look at the latest research on OCD. I will always be grateful to her for assuming a responsibility that I felt my doctors had relinquished. Her name is Catrin and she is married to my close friend Sam Carter.

Psychiatric illnesses fall into two groups: the neuroses and the psychoses, based on whether the patient shows insight into his condition or not. Generally, a neurotic patient will acknowledge that his thoughts and behaviour are abnormal and seek to change them; whereas a patient with psychosis lacks the ability to critically evaluate his thoughts and behaviour as abnormal and in need of modification. Schizophrenia is considered a psychosis and OCD a neurosis. Perhaps this categorisation is better viewed as a spectrum that includes degrees of psychosis and neurosis, as well as the possibility that some of the more bizarre manifestations of a neurosis like OCD could be classified in a hybrid category that blurs the psychosis/neurosis distinction.

These are the highly tentative thoughts of a patient whose only real progress with his neurotic symptoms came when he was treated with medication traditionally prescribed for psychosis. Checking for the squashed bodies of infants on a crowded pavement is certainly neurotic; but looking back from a position where I no longer do that, it strikes me that the extreme irrationality involved was an indicator that insight into my behaviour was so slight that I had breached the borders of neurosis and entered a penumbral phase of my psychiatric regression that contained some of the preliminary elements of psychosis.

The trial period for anti-psychotic augmentation in treatment-resistant OCD is four to six weeks. I have always felt that this intervention enabled me to experience driving in general, and commuting in particular, as a dull necessity that is time lost in the journey of life: rather than a panic spree peppered with multiple incidences of imagined culpable homicide. In all likelihood, that is probably the mundane reality. However, four weeks into my anti-psychotic drug trial period, a very significant shift occurred in my mental response to the obsessions relating to driving.

I was leaving the suburb in which I lived and, shortly after I turned onto the main road leading to the city centre, I passed a cyclist and the usual Obsessive-Compulsive pattern was activated. As I tried to push away the images of being raped in prison once I was convicted, I felt a potent surge of anger. I am certain that the anger was directed at these horrific images that had plagued me for years and at the utter impotence of my attempts to combat them without yielding to the compulsions. I screamed out, "Fuck it! If I am convicted of killing someone accidentally, I will fucking kill myself before anyone can hurt me!"

In that moment I took some control back from the illness. It was the first really effective 'fight or flight' response I had mounted in seven years. All my previous responses had been avoidance tactics – don't drive, avoid public places, stop touching things. These reactions only entrenched and validated the obsessions. The drastic solution proposed in that outburst allowed me to continue the obsession-provoking activity, as well as providing a way to partially neutralise the anxiety. From a psychiatric point of view it was, by definition, a compulsion.

But I had crossed a very dangerous line. That line was the point beyond which suicide became an admissible solution.

You might wonder why I hadn't thought of this before. The acceptability of suicide as a solution to my torment was years in the making and required that the fear of eternity in hell had lost its grip on my psyche. As I understand it, God highly disapproves of a person who predetermines his moment of death. This would suggest that he is not very serious about free will.

Humans can either commit their lives to Jesus or they can go to hell. Most pastors aren't that blunt but any convert-the-masses sermon is really some euphemistic version of this sentiment. Proselytising in this manner insults the notion of free will. Let's call it by its real name: coercion. Coercion is so effective because its power stems from fear. I didn't exercise free will when I became a Christian because I was a scared shitless kid who reacted to the pictures of people burning in hell. It was the only option for me and for millions of Christians around the world who still think that the wages of sin is death. The free will that God so graciously bestowed upon us is of almost no service to human autonomy when there is effectively only one option.

If someone is given the choice between eating a bowl of chocolate mousse and a bowl of faeces, it is ludicrous to suggest that he had made a choice when he tucks into the mousse. And it becomes positively risible to bring choice into the matter if he is told that he will be forced to eat the faeces on Judgement Day unless he becomes a Christian. Christians so often use the free will defence to bolster the image of God as a loving and benevolent creator. I only did undergraduate Philosophy but it was enough for me to establish that the free will referred to by all those Christians boring their secular dinner guests to tears is logically unsound.

I spent years thinking I was either HIV positive or headed for a sodomy-induced death in prison. I didn't want to think about death but I had no choice: I was obsessed with it. I spent a lot of time thinking about religion and the afterlife and, very gradually, settled on atheism as the most rational response to my growing doubts about the irrationalities of many Christian beliefs. Christians have often said to me that it takes more faith to be an atheist than a Christian. Arguing with Christians is almost always futile because they have no intention of altering their beliefs and they are forbidden by God from ever questioning their source material. It is not surprising that this unfalsifiable system of thought has become morally and intellectually stagnant. As Karl Popper noted, unfalsifiable theories are untestable and therefore they cannot evolve in the face of contradictory evidence or improve the veracity of their claims about the world. Atheism requires absolutely no faith. That is the beauty of it.

Once I had thought of suicide and accepted that it was a rational response to my illness, my ability to endure hardship was compromised. It is deeply ironic that my fear of hell had both contributed to my obsessive extrapolations that always ended in death; as well as provided me with some of the capacity to endure the illness of which they were a part. I would never have thought about killing myself while I believed in a literal hell. Suicide became an option in 2002 and all my OCD linked to death - or causing someone else's death - began to fade. There is correlation in this turn of events. Correlation does not imply causation though and the causative variable in this case was probably the anti-psychotic drug Risperdal. I would love to know if my acceptance of suicide as a way out gave Risperdal a helping hand.

It was indeed fortunate that some symptoms of OCD were moderated when suicide and Risperdal were added to my management regime. If suicide had been an option earlier, the temptation to exercise it might have been overwhelming. But OCD has a partner in crime. I didn't meet this partner until a decade after my first round with OCD. I now know why. In my case, he had to wait until suicide became an option because the way he hurts his victims is to play with their minds and emotions until some of them kill themselves. He doesn't always succeed; but anyone who has tried to fight him off for long enough will tell you that in the darkest moments, suicidal impulses are a source of comfort rather than horror.

Chapter VIII

Perhaps Sweden would've helped

In January 1995, on our way back to Zimbabwe from our holiday in Cape Town, I stopped over in Johannesburg to stay with my friend Sam Carter while my family continued up to Harare. Sam was the first person I told about what was happening to me.

We had met when we were kids while his family was living in Zimbabwe. They left Zimbabwe because his father had a PhD in engineering and was under-employed in the country's unsophisticated economy. Johannesburg offered more fulfilling and better paid work and so, when Sam and I were eleven, the Carter family emigrated to South Africa. We stayed in contact over the years; and, despite our different personalities, we always had a strong friendship that we would consolidate whenever they were in Harare or we were in Johannesburg. Sam introduced me to books and British humour for which I am particularly grateful. I tried to get him to lift weights which he rejected out of hand, I think, because his overriding goal in life was to develop his mind. He could see no point in the ability to bench press anything other than his duvet on a hot night.

Sam left the Church earlier than I did but his was an intellectual decision; while I strayed from the flock because of my inability to conquer a deadly sin. Sam wrote a philosophical tract at the tender age of seventeen, laying out the reasons for his self-imposed excommunication. He read it to me while I was still a Christian and I found it to be impressively compelling. I didn't understand all of it but I recall that, in essence, he said that he was sick of feeling guilty all the time.

I could relate to that but I was not as brave as he was at that age. I am now of the opinion that if God is serious about reforming his notion of free will, then he has to concede that renouncing Christianity cannot be a punishable offence. I don't think Sam was sure of this reality which is why he was so brave at the time. I, on the other hand, was still convinced that a literal hell was the punishment for absence of faith and so - although I was tempted to join my friend in the peaceful glade of atheism - I was too terrified of brimstone baths and burnt flesh to take the step.

It occurs to me that some Christians reading this book will see my OCD as punishment from God for rejecting religion; and might even go as far as to say that I got what was coming to me as a sinner under the Devil's command. They might even believe that my Obsessive-Compulsive bondage was evidence that I was possessed by demons and that only when my illness leads me back to the Lord will I be delivered from my torment. I have thought all these things and worse; and have in fact returned to the Church and Christianity on four occasions since the first withdrawal in 1994. As recently as 2005 I was born again, again; and shortly thereafter I was told by a fiery prophet from Cameroon, that the Devil would have no power over me and that my face would shine with glory. Actually, the fellow could only speak French and it was his translator who uttered these encouraging remarks. I don't speak French, so it's possible that the translator was protecting me from a more disheartening set of predictions. For all I know the prophet was saying, "This guy's future looks pretty grim. God does not believe that OCD is a real illness and would like it very much if Andrew would pull himself together. Satan seems to be pleased at the high cost of psychiatric drugs and will ensure that Andrew never takes generic medicine. Oh dear, this poor fellow."

Whatever he said, he might have served me better if he had dispensed with the unfalsifiable generalities and warned me that six months later I would almost succeed in killing myself.

During my stay with Sam in Johannesburg in January 1995, we went out to a bar. Having a few too many is an excellent way for friends to deepen their bonds and that night was no different. We stumbled home after a respectable number of pints and were noisily slurping the tea we had brewed in the hope of nipping our oncoming hangovers in the bud, when I said to Sam:

"This is gonna sound weird, but on the way back from the bar I was looking over my shoulder to see if I had stepped on a baby."
"What are you talking about?"
"I have been doing it for a month now. Since December. I can't stop."
"Are you joking - And? Perhaps we should talk about this when we've sobered up."
"I haven't told anyone except you. It's fuckin' crazy."
"This is freaking me out. You need to talk to someone – maybe a doctor – about this. I think we should go to bed and think about it tomorrow."

I remember that I used a jocular tone, attempting to lessen the impact of what was in reality a shocking revelation. I didn't tell him about any of the other symptoms although, in our inebriated stupor, I'm not sure that Sam had any idea how to respond to even that one neurotic morsel. We didn't talk about it the next day. I imagine that Sam's very rational mind forgot about the whole thing until the events that unfolded two months later.

Fly Fishing For Sharks

I travelled back to Harare in mid-January with my cousin and my aunt. On the morning we left I was unusually besieged by obsessions about babies and blood. As we crested a rise on the busy motorway I looked out over the city and wondered if anyone of those millions of people was experiencing what was happening to me. I didn't know that I had a recognised illness and had never heard of anything even remotely similar to my experience. As I tried to avoid letting my skin touch the upholstery of the car's back seat, deriving no solace from the fact that it was a brand spanking new vehicle, I felt utterly alone.

The journey from Johannesburg to Harare is more than a thousand kilometres long. There are no noteworthy towns along the way; the scenery is quite bland and there is a needless waste of time at the shabby Beitbridge border post just north of Messina - the town where *apartheid* had still been alive and well in 1993 and where African athleticism had triumphed over Afrikaans thuggery. For an Obsessive-Compulsive with contamination issues, this border post is purgatory. Most people passing through Beitbridge are either walking across in the sweltering heat or crammed into dilapidated buses and taxis that are life-threateningly unroadworthy. I am irrationally afraid of mass poverty, not least because I fear ending up that way but also because I feel that if I were them, I would resent the relative affluence of others.

That day at the border post I was even more obsessed than usual about stepping on a baby because I was white and all the poor people were black. I was bombarded with vivid mental images of being beaten to death by an enraged mob, a mob who would see me not only as a murderer but also as a killer driven by racism to squash a defenceless child to death. It was all going pretty badly in my mind. Then I went to the toilets on the Zimbabwean side and the real trouble started. They hadn't been cleaned for weeks and there was no toilet paper in sight. Of course, there were no visible signs of blood but the stench of urine and sight of excrement were so repulsive to me that it was days before I had even partial relief from the persistent suspicion that I was now HIV positive.

As we drove north to Harare, I began to indulge in some counterfactual speculation about whether I would have developed such bizarre psychopathology if I had lived in Europe - and particularly Sweden. My grandfather was Swedish. He came to Africa seeking opportunity and an escape from the harsh winters of Scandinavia. Rhodesia, as it was then known, offered him the chance to live in a frontier society where resolute entrepreneurs with a stomach for risk could find their place in the sun. Twenty-first century Sweden is a prosperous welfare state with minimal poverty and high living standards whose citizens are, on the whole probably safer and better educated than most of humanity. But the Sweden of the early 1900s did not offer a very high standard of living to many of its citizens.

My grandfather did not plan to go back to Sweden, going so far as renouncing his right to Swedish citizenship when the time came to choose. When Zimbabwe began to show signs of implosion in 2000 and the Alexander family faced the dilemma of where to emigrate, we began to regret that we had no ancestral rights to Swedish citizenship, which would have carried the added benefit of a European Union passport. Our other European ancestors had arrived in Africa from Britain a couple of generations too early to make any difference. It turned out that our only choice was South Africa and, compared to most Zimbabweans, we were extremely lucky to have even that one option.

My speculation about my Swedish ancestry and its associated 'what ifs' relates to what psychiatry calls psychosocial stress. As I understand it, psychosocial stress is a blanket term for all exogenous or environmental factors that might exacerbate an illness. Crudely speaking, a person with a phobia about dirt might function better in Switzerland than he would in Calcutta; and a person abnormally concerned about his personal safety might prefer to be posted to rural Denmark than he would be to present-day Baghdad.

I have never been to Sweden but I have read enough issues of the *Economist*, various *National Geographic* articles and almanacs to know that it is a place vastly different to Zimbabwe. To begin with, Swedes tend to be more relaxed about sexuality than Zimbabweans. If I had been discovered on a quest to explore my pre-adolescent sexuality by Swedish parents, they might have sat me down and patiently explained to me that my curiosity was natural but that I needed to wait a couple of years before I tried that again. Heck, if they had been really liberated, they might have patted me on the back for early-onset virility, lovingly mentioning that other parents would not see it that way; and then suggested that it would be wise to concentrate for now on my soccer or ice hockey.

I once asked a Scandinavian whether she knew of any 'happy clapper' churches in her part of the world and - once I had explained the unfamiliar term to her - she replied that maybe they existed but she did not know of any. I understand that the State Church in Sweden is influential in politics and that many Swedes are paid-up members; but I am also led to believe that Sweden is a predominantly secular society, where the concept of a literal hell of fire and brimstone is understood in the popular consciousness to be about as valid as the lost city of Atlantis or Medusa's snake bouffant. If this is even partially correct, it seems unlikely that I would have been to teenage camps in Sweden at which vulnerable adolescents were told that the wages of sin is death, or that masturbation with lustful thoughts is wrong. On the contrary, I would have had access to some of the world's finest pornography and - if I was good looking - one or two Swedish girlfriends who knew that sex did not result in babies or AIDS if you were equipped with condoms and birth control pills.

Without an irrational fear of hell and a moral framework that assessed actions according to their consequences, not on whether or not Big Brother approved, I might never have become so obsessed with death and my own indelible sinfulness. My theory of morality was revolutionised by the observation Sam Harris made in his book, *The End of Faith,* that many of what the Bible calls sins are victimless crimes. I think people like Deuteronomy, the camp leader, would do the world a favour if they took that observation into consideration before they told teenage boys surging with already confusing hormones that sexual fantasies are wrong or that masturbation combined with sexual thoughts is offensive to God.

However, if OCD is caused by a combination of genetic and environmental factors - as scientists propose - then not even safe, clean and prosperous Sweden would have prevented the emergence of the illness at some stage of my life. What forms it would have taken I don't know, but I have always enjoyed counterfactual speculation and I can't resist applying it to the dominant force in my life. Earlier, I mentioned that I described OCD as 'the tyranny of what ifs', so, at the risk of joining dots that are not there, it is perhaps unsurprising that I am so intrigued by counterfactual exercises.

Chapter IX

In need of more serotonin

I don't have very clear memories of the weeks before my first breakdown because I was preoccupied with the fact that 'A' level examination results were due out in early February. OCD continued to be terrifying but I was hanging on because I had convinced myself that the symptoms would clear up once I got to UCT - a state of mind that I imagine derived from a belief that the bizarre obsessions had arisen during the stressful examination period when I was aware that my future hung in the balance.

This conviction was bolstered by the naïve notion that South Africa was more like a first world country, thus there OCD would not be a problem. The attendant equanimity not only related to the fears of contamination and killing people. I also thought that the OCD I battled with academically could be neutralised with as yet untapped seams of willpower. It was almost as if I thought South Africa seemed to offer the same protection from my nightmare that I assumed would exist in Sweden.

I am, of course, applying the term OCD retrospectively to my memories. At that stage I still had no idea of the illness's chronic course or even that I was ill. I really did believe that I was at risk of contracting AIDS or killing someone accidentally and viewed my compulsions as necessary vigilance. What is quite interesting to note is that, after diagnosis, I assumed that I would have more control over my behaviour and thoughts; erroneously anticipating that because I could attribute the symptoms to a recognised illness, they would decrease in frequency and intensity.

Within hours of word going out that the 'A' level results had arrived from England, young men and women gathered at the schools that they had left at the end of 1994 and waited in line to receive the little slip of paper that could make or break their futures. You will remember that I had had to write my exams at two schools because of the OCD-related problems. I thus had to pick up two sets of results at separate locations; and take a double hit of the frayed nerves syndrome that sets in before you unfold the results sheet and see how you did. I was most concerned about my Mathematics result because a decent pass was needed to gain acceptance to the finance degree that I intended to take at UCT.

To my utter amazement I got an 'A' for Geography but I put that down to the fact that I wrote three of the four essays in the exam on climate and weather, subjects that were a hobby of mine. For English, I got a 'B' because of my low scores on the Shakespeare paper but that was not surprising. Thank Baal for Mrs Davidson - my private tutor - and my mother's intervention because I have little doubt that if I had soldiered on with Dickens, Hardy and Austen, I would have got an 'E'- or worse.

I failed Maths. This was devastating but considering that I had spent one third of the exam engaged in pointless checking and another third fighting the obsession about the cyclist I might have hit, it was only to be expected. I phoned the university to ask them what the implications were for my choice of degree and I was ecstatic to find out that if I had a 'B' grade or higher in Additional Maths, I could still register for the finance programme. Additional Maths was more difficult than 'O' level but not as hard as 'A' level; and I had taken the subject in my fourth year at high school before OCD became too severe. I had achieved a 'B' grade which meant that my Wall Street dream did not have to be shelved just yet.

Career dreams tend to exhibit grandiose reckonings of an individual's talent and an inappropriate disregard for the obstacles that stand in the way of a successful realisation. These characteristics are particularly acute when the chosen career path leads to fame or fortune. This quixotic stance is needed to buffer people against setbacks and sustain ambition. No-one goes to Hollywood or New York with a burning desire to become a waiter unless they want a fairly muted farewell party. And yet, most aspirant actors and millionaires find employment that offers insignificance and penury. I bet there are cleaning staff on Wall Street with better Maths records than I had: you see what I mean about grandiose reckonings and disregard for obstacles – *quod erat demonstrandum* indeed.

Over the following two weeks, I prepared to leave OCD and Zimbabwe behind me for good. Plane tickets were booked, study visas were secured and bags were packed as most of my good friends and I got ready for university and a new life in Cape Town. On the morning I was scheduled to leave, I sat down beside my mother's bed and, while we sipped our traditional cups of morning tea, I said to her in a tremulous voice, "Do you think I will be able to cope at university?" Years later, she recounted to me that she had been very surprised by my question because she knew that I had wanted to go to UCT ever since I knew what university was.

The plane trip down to Cape Town was so exciting that I didn't worry too much about looking over my shoulder for babies as I walked across the tarmac towards the aeroplane at Harare International Airport; or as I walked through Johannesburg airport to catch my connecting flight to Cape Town.

In hindsight, that was the first sign of real trouble. Both flights were full of Zimbabwean students and there was such an air of anticipation that I delayed the inevitable realisation that I was just as bad in South Africa - a delay driven by a vague premonition that my life, my future and everything I held dear would be destroyed once I did. I was in denial and it was working. I now know that the longer you stay in denial, the more you jeopardise the eventual acceptance that is the start of real progress and the only source of true healing.

The first week was orientation and wine, women and song – well, not really, it was beer and song and - for most of us - a disappointing lack of women. It quickly became clear that there was a roughly even split between women and men on campus and the seven-to-one ratio altered its status from godsend to dead end in a mere seventy-two hours. Like tourists on safari, we were continually on the lookout for the horny male's big five – breasts, bum, legs, hair and face. Cape Town did not disappoint. On campus, at the nightclubs and especially on the beach, we spotted Helen of Troy after Helen of Troy and, although in classical mythology she was reported to have a face that launched one thousand ships, here each heavenly Helen produced at least that many erections on an average day in public. We speculated that inanimate wooden boats would not respond to beauty but that, in ancient Greece, 'ship' must have been a metaphor for 'penis'.

The beginning of the collapse started on the first day of lectures. My anxiety had spiked the night before, when a senior in our residence had made threatening gestures at me and this hastened the disintegration of my denial. The contamination fears were especially bad in the dining hall and the public bathrooms; and the baby obsession became more acute. I did not have a car in Cape Town, thus driving was not a problem; but the shock of coming to terms with the fact that OCD had followed me to Cape Town was too much of a blow to my coping responses.

I remember getting off the bus on the first day of classes and walking along the patterned bricking of the University's main thoroughfare, my mind flooded with images of dead babies. Being on public transport for the first time had fuelled my contamination fears. In the first lecture, academic OCD came flooding back and I missed most of the notes from the overhead projector because I was compulsively re-reading what I had begun to copy down. I quickly descended to the point where I was checking the chair I was about to sit on for blood; and then for dead babies when I stood up to leave the lecture hall. Not only did I think I might have stood on one as I walked around, I now thought I might sit on one and suffocate it to death.

The Maths lecture sparked the same dysfunctionality I had battled with in my 'A' level years and I had to admit to myself that eventual failure of the course was inevitable, with even the most optimistic projection of my ability to control further deterioration.

The following few days saw a rapid decline in my state of mind. The obsessions were out of control and - difficult though it was to admit - I was acutely aware of one irrefutable fact: something was gravely wrong and I was not going to last much longer. I decided, after crying for about an hour in the toilet with the toilet seat covered in toilet paper to protect me from blood, to ask for help for the first time since the missing swearword scenario three years previously. Fortunately, we had many family friends in Cape Town so I just needed to pick one. I chose a deeply spiritual and compassionate lady called Jane Hulley.

It might seem incongruous that I chose someone spiritual, given my distaste for religion but, like many people, I make a firm distinction between people who are spiritual and those who are religious. Spirituality is possible without any formal religious beliefs. However, I am deeply suspicious of people who tell me that they are spiritual beings in the same way that self-proclaimed intellectuals are often nothing of the sort. Spirituality takes years to attain and, as with all attainments, it is better to have others confirm your status than it is to decide for yourself.

I have often found that spiritual people are compassionate in ways that religious people can only dream of. Religious people too often see the world in terms of Them and Us and the disapproval they extend to so many segments of society has the effect of curtailing their capacity for compassion. A religious fellow named Victor once called me an "enemy of God," an epithet I disregarded after he told a friend of mine that Mozart and Beethoven's music was tainted with the devil because they were not born-again Christians. If I am an "enemy of God", I wonder whether it would influence Victor's behaviour if I really needed his help. For Jane it wouldn't matter, it would be enough that I was a human who was suffering in some way. That is why I describe her as spiritual.

Jane's family had been our neighbours in my childhood Capetonian suburb of Llandudno: and her son and I had watched *Mia the Bee* together as four-year-olds. I phoned her and said that something was wrong. I asked her if she could come and pick me up and take me to her house so that I could phone my parents. The phones in my residence were in a very public place and I was worried that I would break down in front of everyone. Jane gave me dinner and asked what was wrong but I was too confused and frightened to give her any details. At first she suspected homesickness but during the course of the evening her intuition told her that something more sinister was at work.

Fly Fishing For Sharks

After dinner, I went upstairs to the Hulleys' study and closed the door to ensure that no-one in the house heard what was likely to be a terrible conversation. My mother answered the phone in Harare, surprised to hear from me. She was also in somewhat of a rush because she was accompanying my father to a business function and they were running late. In a deeply strained tone I tried to give her a synopsis of what was happening to me but my mouth was dry from the anxiety and I was particularly incoherent – no doubt because I had so much to say and so little time.

"Mom, hi, it's Andrew."

"Hi darling, I'm sorry I can't speak for long because dad and I are going to a Coopers function."

"Mom....um....I am phoning from Jane Hulley's house. Things aren't going very well."

"What do you mean? You seemed fine the other day."

"I know but I was hoping it would go away."

"What are you talking about?"

"I get these horrible thoughts, mom – scary thoughts. It got worse down here, but I wanted to come to UCT."

"What do you mean it got worse? Worse than what? Andrew, can you tell me what's actually wrong."

"I think it is para....noid del...usion..al psy...psychosis."

"I can't hear what you are saying, darling."

"Sorry my mouth is very dry from being nervous. It's not easy to talk."

"Andrew, dad and I are very late. Do you want to phone us tomorrow when there is more time?"

"Mom, I need to come home. I'm very ill."

"I'm sure that is the not best option. Are you sure you're not just overwhelmed by your new environment, and feeling homesick?"

"Please, mom, believe me that I am in trouble."

"Well, Frank's wedding is in Jo'burg on Saturday. Fly up tomorrow and we can discuss this over the weekend. We'll meet you at the Carters tomorrow evening."

"Mom, how do I book a ticket?"

"Andrew, if you can't organise a ticket, something must be really wrong with you."

"Sorry, mom, I just can't think str...straight. Please don't be cross."

"Get Jane to help you. We really have to go. We'll see you tomorrow."

"Thanks mom, bye."

"Bye."

I had told her that I had "paranoid delusional psychosis" but I had not the faintest idea what that meant. It was a description I picked up from the movie *Ace Ventura: Pet Detective*. Aren't Hollywood screenplays just so useful in life's trickier moments? It had been used by Jim Carrey's character when describing an obviously insane woman he encountered during his investigation into the source of a series of death threats targeting a football player whose team mascot had been kidnapped – I think it was a dolphin - which is why they needed Ace.

Not many parents like the sound of paranoid delusional psychosis and my mother was no different. Her fear came across as anger in the comment, "Something must be really wrong with you." I don't hold it against her but it did confirm one of my most isolating concerns: namely that no-one would be able to relate to what I was going through and therefore that I was unlikely to receive much empathy – empathy that would be vital to finding help. I felt like a terrified child who loses his parents in a crowd and that abysmal sense of aloneness that I had experienced on the busy highway in Johannesburg returned. My mother has been the most steadfast and committed member of my support network but that evening I felt like an orphan.

Jane was like a mother that night in February 1995; and, sensing that I was desperate, she sprang into action and booked me a flight, paid for it and arranged for her son to take me to the airport in the morning. She dropped me back at my residence and I went up to my room to pack a small bag of clothes to see myself through the weekend.

My room-mate was a good friend of mine named Steven Saffin. He knew that I was not coping although he was a little unsure about how to respond to a guy who had been putting on a brave face and entertaining his friends as recently as orientation week. It is amazing what a powerful coping strategy denial is. We can present as happy and normal in the midst of a crisis to the extent that we believe it will all soon be over. As soon as denial reaches the limits of its adaptive capacity, the subsequent collapse is sometimes astonishingly rapid. In four days I had gone from thinking that I could handle my problems to a childlike helplessness.

I didn't tell Steven about the bizarre thoughts. I just told him that I was going to Johannesburg for a wedding. We spent the evening listening to Bon Jovi while he entertained me with his amazing capacity to comment intelligently on an impressive variety of topics. I could hardly concentrate but the distraction of his lengthy conversational opinion pieces was just what I needed that night. I mention Bon Jovi because they wrote a song called *Without Love* that gave me hope amidst the turmoil that night. One of the lines is: "There is nothing without love, and nothing else will get you through the night." I still don't know exactly why that song meant so much to me but I think that the experience of an uplifting emotion was so powerful that evening because all the other feelings and thoughts inside of me were terrifying.

A curious thing about OCD that I have observed is that it always intensifies when I know I am going to get help or when I am preparing to leave a place in which a major relapse has occurred. The morning I left UCT for Johannesburg was my first experience of this aspect of the illness. Jane Hulley's son, Alexander, was due to take me to the airport and his flat was a mere two blocks from my residence building. As I walked out of my room with my small bag of clothes slung over my shoulder, the obsessions surged to their highest-ever level of intensity. I managed to get half way down the corridor before I felt forced to return to my room and check everywhere for dead babies.

I took about twenty minutes to walk three hundred metres to the door of his apartment. Previously, I had been able to glance over my shoulder while continuing to walk; but that morning I had to stop about every ten metres, turn around and scan the pavement in a ritualistic manner that involved repeatedly moving my head up and down as I sought to confirm the fact that my eyes were covering every inch of the unchecked pavement. Other pedestrians must have believed they were witnessing the behaviour of an insane individual who had been given a day pass from the psychiatric facility not far from the university.

If someone faints on a sidewalk or a blind person is having difficulty finding his way, it is human nature to feel pity for that person and offer some assistance. If an obviously insane person makes an appearance in public and exhibits signs of distress, however, it is human nature to feel revulsion and avoid eye contact or any form of engagement. The escaped madman is one of society's most lurid avatars of the risk posed to its members by those elements we consider dangerous. This revulsion and misunderstanding directed towards the mentally ill is a source of the estrangement that sufferers like me feel and a cause of the intense shame that so hinders our assertiveness and thwarts our recovery.

According to the *Economist*, 50 per cent of media coverage devoted to the mentally ill deals with those of us who commit acts of violence. Statistically, only 3 per cent of the mentally ill are violent towards others and that figure is no higher than the one for the general population. Psychiatrists will tell you that on average, an individual's proclivity for violence existed prior to the onset of the illness, after which the expression of this tendency became more bizarre and unpredictable. Admittedly, murders committed by the mentally ill do sell newspapers for this reason. While I am happy to concede the saleability of stories dealing with crimes committed by the mentally ill, it must be remembered that this does not alter the very low statistical likelihood of their occurrence. Because of the horrors of mental illness, sufferers sometimes kill themselves. A contributing factor is how badly they are handled by their support networks and society at large. Society has more blood on its hands than the mentally ill. Mental illnesses themselves are responsible for only a negligible percentage of the violence that humans visit on each other.

The first time that morning that I had any respite from the torment was when I sat down in my window seat on the plane. As the plane banked north, I looked out of the window and could see the UCT campus on the slopes of Table Mountain. I could quite clearly identify the cylindrical residence block where I had slept the night before. My room number was 518 and it still held most of my worldly possessions. Although I had no idea what awaited me in Johannesburg, I was adamant that I would not see the cheap metallic numbers on its door ever again. I was so desperate to get help that I had no emotional space to feel disappointment.

As I looked out through the aeroplane window, I remembered a haunting photograph I'd seen in a *National Geographic* article on refugees of an Asian girl being flown to safety in America. The picture was taken from outside the plane and through the rain-splattered window the photographer had captured the face of a terrified and tearful human being. I began to sob. It was what a fellow patient in my first psychiatric ward had called 'a soul cry'. He said that when grown men truly cry, it is their soul that is weeping. The passengers next to me could see that I was inconsolable and they reached out indirectly by communicating to the air hostess on my behalf when the meal was served. Try as I might, I was unable to speak through the tears. I indicated what I wanted to eat and drink by nodding or shaking my head as they listed the options.

Sam Carter's mother, Di, and Rob, his brother, picked me up in Johannesburg and drove me to their house where my parents were due to arrive from Zimbabwe later that afternoon. I told them that something was seriously wrong with me but I didn't go into details. I lay down on Sam's bed exhausted, hoping to get some sleep. I felt safe for the first time in a long while but I was too upset to fall asleep.

Wordsworth called sleep "the poor man's wealth" and, since the beginning of the illness, I have sought refuge in sleep although anxiety and horrible thoughts have often delayed the onset of a restful slumber. OCD has featured in my dreams only twice in all the years that I have been living with it. I am blessed with the gift of uninterrupted and restorative sleep that is almost never disturbed by nightmares. My subconscious is up against formidable competition because, on many days, OCD is a living nightmare and anything that my subconscious could produce would have to push the envelope of terror to frighten me. The one drawback of sleep is that you have to wake up every morning. When I feel suicidal, the comfort I derive from such a grim emotion is that if I succeed in killing myself, I will never have to wake up. Morbid though it may sound, there have been times when that concept has almost been a fantasy.

Acting on a tip-off from Di that I was in bad shape, my parents arrived and took me straight off to a hotel where they booked me my own room. We had a quiet dinner and made plans to see a doctor in the morning. The first doctor I saw was a GP. She stopped me in the middle of my story to say that she had briefly studied my condition in medical school but was not sufficiently qualified to deal with my case. She phoned a psychiatrist at a private psychiatric hospital and arranged an appointment for that afternoon.

We met him in an observation room where he asked me to give an account of my problems, and I spoke continuously for half an hour. As I described my world, my mother began to cry.

The psychiatrist, who was obviously a gifted note-taker, filled page after page with what seemed like every word I said. When I had finished he put down his pen, paused for a moment or two and then calmly said that I had an illness called Obsessive-Compulsive Disorder that was caused by an imbalance of a neurotransmitter called serotonin in my synaptic clefts and, as luck would have it, a new drug called Prozac was now available to treat the symptoms. He wanted to admit me to the psychiatric ward for three weeks where he would be able to monitor my progress on Prozac which he wanted me to begin taking immediately. All my worst prejudices about mental institutions provoked a strong reaction to his suggestion and I politely refused to be admitted. He asked if we had any close and supportive family friends in town who would be able to look after me during the early weeks of treatment. In a fit of relief, both my mother and I quickly blurted out in unison, "the Carters."

The doctor asked for details and - once he was satisfied that they were up to the task - he agreed that I could stay with them, provided they committed to driving me to his rooms twice a week so that he could monitor possible side effects of the medication and assess any progress with regard to my symptom profile.

The diagnosis was on the Friday in the last week of February 1995. After my cousin's wedding that weekend my parents returned to Harare to get back to work and give the news to my brother and sister. I waved goodbye to them in the early hours of Monday morning with Di Carter standing next to me wondering, I imagine, how on earth she was going to look after four boys, her beloved husband and the very ill teenager who had been entrusted to her care for three weeks. Di Carter is a beautiful woman with the perfect balance of femininity and fortitude. She probably didn't feel very confident that morning but she turned out to be the perfect candidate for the job at hand. She now lives in America with her husband Pete, but the whole Carter family are still some of the most important people in my life.

Chapter X

At least I haven't contracted the Ebola virus

I spent just over three weeks at the Carter's house; and twice a week Di drove me to the psychiatrist for check-ups. None of the symptoms were alleviated but I derived great relief from knowing that what I had experienced had a name; and that it was theoretically treatable. In addition, I was under almost no stress. Throughout my illness, extreme stress has been an irritatingly dependable predictor and cause of relapse.

I spent most of the days indoors in front of the television or reading books. The Carters are one of the most well-read families I know and their house was full of excellent books. Although my reading was still marred by compulsive repetition, this hassle was attenuated by the fact that I had all the time in the world; as well as the euphoric realisation that almost every book in the world was less difficult to read than *Bleak House* by Charles Dickens.

I remember reading a book entitled *The Hot Zone* that dealt with the unimaginable horrors of the Ebola virus and a few other gruesome tropical diseases. This was a spectacularly poor choice of reading matter on my part. With a morbid obsession about being infected with AIDS, I should have avoided a non-fiction title about viruses that make AIDS seem comparatively benign. Within pages the old obsession about the stalker with his syringe of HIV-positive blood reared its head again and evolved into a scenario in which his syringe was a vector of the Ebola virus.

By the second day, I was covering my glasses of milk with napkins in case he was squirting the Ebola virus through miniscule holes in the ceiling that he had quietly bored with the needle of his syringe. I stood on chairs to scrutinise large sections of imperforated white ceiling boards for telltale signs of needles sticking through, aimed at my glass of milk. This behaviour persisted for a few days after I decided that *The Hot Zone* was unwise reading but thankfully the obsession did not become chronic like so many of the others.

Perhaps influenced by the optimistic prognosis of the psychiatrist, my mother had already booked me a return flight to Cape Town and arranged for UCT to hold my room in residence and maintain my registration for the finance degree. By week three, I realised that this anticipated return to study was not possible that year and that I would probably return to Zimbabwe to live at home and continue my treatment. I was too frightened of the outside world to be disappointed at this reality and considered my return to the country I was so desperate to leave preferable to the prospect of trying to cope on my own at university. Disappointment would have to take a back seat to the overriding drive to avoid the anxiety-provoking situations that became the *sine qua non* of my existence after diagnosis. I invested a lot of hope in the green and white capsules I now swallowed every night. Losing hope was one of the most emotionally debilitating experiences of my battle with OCD and it heralded the arrival of OCD's partner in crime and my struggle with suicidal thoughts and behaviour.

In an earlier chapter I mentioned, in passing, OCD's partner in crime. Let me now introduce you properly. His name is Depression. OCD and Major Depression exhibit a strong co-morbid relationship. OCD usually precedes the onset of Major Depression but the cruel reality of this partnership is that the activation of Depression is, in many cases, associated with almost no amelioration of the symptoms of OCD. In fact the power of Major Depression to render you helpless means that your ability to cope with OCD is diminished further and this can make it seem worse than before.

I am concerned that people reading this book will think that in an attempt to do justice to the trauma of the illness, I have given myself the license to exaggerate. I note, with apprehension, the emotionally charged adjectives, adverbs and intensifiers that recur, perhaps too frequently, in sections of the book in which I describe the onset or recurrence of symptoms. In particular, the expression 'Major Depression' might appear to have the colloquial embellishment so often observed in the unsolicited litanies of very minor crises that teenage drama queens – and kings for that matter – never tire of inflicting on their friends. This is a strategy for validation that I do not want to employ.

My experiences with mental illness may have been less traumatic for other men and women of more heroic constitutions. But as I trawl through my memories and put them on paper, I am aware that although I was equipped with a certain quota of emotional, mental and physical strength, on many occasions over the years my illness was stronger than my ability to cope. When I remember those occasions now, I feel that it is no exaggeration to say that they were truly horrible. As this is a memoir, that assessment of the dark days is necessarily subjective.

I called it 'Major Depression' because that is what the psychiatrists call depression that is affecting the patient's functionality to a severe extent. It is so called to distinguish it from 'Minor Depression' which has a less restrictive effect on functionality. It is worth bearing in mind, though, that even Minor Depression is a very major pain in the rear. Teenage drama queens have three or four major crises a day and they are usually exaggerating; but in the world of mental illness, 'major' is just an indication of degree. For those who have experienced the helplessness of Depression, the word 'major' is something of an understatement.

'Catastrophic Depression' comes closer to the devastated lives that this illness leaves in its wake. 'Depression', 'depressing' and 'depressed' are words used every day by all sorts of people to describe a temporary lowering of mood; or to account for a reaction to some stimulus that has made them sad. People often say they get depressed on a Sunday night in anticipation of going to work the next day. If you feel a bit down and are restored by a warm bath and a re-run of your favourite movie, then you are not depressed in a clinical sense. If you are emotionally obliterated by the thought of your job, lose your appetite, wake up anxious at four in the morning and can't go back to sleep and, in extreme cases, consider ending your life rather than getting up the next day, then depressed is an accurate word for how you are feeling. The overuse of the word 'Depression' has diluted its meaning and contributed to the lack of empathy exhibited by many people towards those who are clinically depressed.

I think the reason for this overuse is that - like so many psychiatric conditions - Depression is a spectrum disorder. A severe case is characterised by the presence of extreme examples of emotions and thought processes that, further back along the spectrum, are experienced by almost everyone. Type 1 Diabetes is not a spectrum disorder because you either have it or you don't. Diabetic comas are distinct medical phenomena and so you don't often hear a healthy person lie back on the couch after a hard day and say, "You know, honey, I am having a partial diabetic coma, please inject me with a dilute solution of insulin." As a spectrum disorder, Depression is different because everyone has travelled some way down the slippery slope to meltdown at the hands of clinical depression.

Fly Fishing For Sharks

Clinical Depression is a neurochemical illness that gives the sufferer about as much control over his symptoms as an epileptic. You would not say "pull yourself together" to an individual writhing on the floor in the middle of a grand mal seizure. The visual reality of the symptoms would frighten you into action and you would do what you could to help the sufferer. Just because the symptoms of clinical Depression are not visible, it does not render them any less real or debilitating.

The mentally ill are largely rejected by the communities they need the most. I attribute this to the fact that, in many cases, the symptoms are not visible and it is difficult to imagine what the sufferer is going through. If you wouldn't tell an epileptic having a fit to "pull himself together", then you should not try that line on a psychiatric patient just because your eyes can't tell you anything about his pain. Rather, and especially if the person is close to you, say, "I feel helpless and scared because I don't know how to help you."

A psychiatrist once said to me after a very serious suicide attempt, "Andrew, what you really need now is courage." I had had about ten stitches in each wrist and there was dried blood all over my stomach and legs. I had used all my courage slicing those deep cuts in my wrists and was in no mood for an expensive pep talk. If I had been feeling strong at the time, I would have said, "What I need is science and medicine. This isn't the Battle of Agincourt and you're not Henry V. Now stop cheerleading and act like a doctor."

Humans are a highly developed species that is the product of hundreds of millions of years of evolution but we are eons away from the status of morally sophisticated organisms. The single most powerful restraint on human behaviour is fear: fear of punishment, fear of God, fear of hell, fear of guilt. This is an unsound basis for moral development. Until we behave ethically for the simple reason that the thing we are about to do is wrong in and of itself, we are not much better than a criminal whose only reason for not committing crimes is the impenetrable fortress of his maximum security cell.

I realised that I wasn't an intellectual when I read Kant's seminal text, *The Critique of Pure Reason*, in undergraduate Philosophy. In fact, I had some inkling that I wasn't an intellectual when I wrote a scholarship exam for high school and prayed for divine inspiration in the Maths paper. Whatever number popped into my head was the answer I gave. I defy anyone to finish Kant's book with their self-image in one piece. Kant's Golden Rule was that we should treat people as ends in themselves rather than as means to an end. If we treat our own attempts at a moral existence as an end in itself, we can appreciate that one implication of widening the scope of Kant's principle is that a person achieves true morality only when he does the right thing without the stick of punishment or the carrot of reward.

The extension of Kant's principle to encompass morality as a whole is obviously an ideal; but, if the moral capacity of our species evolved towards that ideal, the theoretical removal of the mechanisms of social control would become immaterial. As born-again Kantians, we wouldn't need anticipation of reward or fear of punishment to do the right thing. Establishing right from wrong would no doubt remain a complicated process; but ethical debate would benefit from the removal of the largely black or white thinking of religious participants. Atheism, on the other hand, is no barrier to ethical behaviour and morality's shift to a secular paradigm would allow brilliant people like Richard Dawkins a destigmatised voice on a range of issues outside the scope of the Ten Commandments. The Vatican's stance on birth control is a good example of how the continued and unquestioning referencing of ancient documents can lead to unnecessary suffering and moral irrelevance. Sadly, I think that there is an outside chance that religious fundamentalism will catalyse humanity's demise well before evolution produces the first *Homo sapiens kantus*.

The second term that I introduced – 'co-morbid' – requires much less explaining than 'depression'. It is just another medical term to describe a patient who is experiencing the symptoms of two distinct illnesses whose relationship is causative. In my case, I am identified by my long-suffering medical insurance company as having 'treatment-resistant Obsessive-Compulsive Disorder with co-morbid Major Depression'. The company covers the unforeseen costs associated with my psychiatric instability; and have paid out considerably more money than my similarly long-suffering father has kindly paid in on my behalf over the years. The company must regret the day it agreed to insure me but its liabilities are an inevitable feature of an industry engaged in sophisticated risk analysis of events in an unknowable future.

Chapter XI

University – Take 2

A young man returning home from University four years early to a small community like ours in Harare is bound to be the stuff of rumours. People who knew me- and people who knew of me - must have talked; but I heard very little of it. I tried to be as open as possible but when you start talking about stepping on babies, very few people go away thinking, "Oh well, that's all right then."

I would describe myself now as an 'overconfessor' – a clumsy neologism if there ever was one. After years of being incoherent and evasive when someone said, "What do you do?", one day I thought, "Screw it, I'm mentally ill and I'm proud" and decided that henceforth I would tell people that there was good reason that I lived at home and received an allowance. This candid approach and a growing sense that I had no reason to feel ashamed probably laid some of the psychological groundwork for writing this book.

There is very little to say about that year back in Harare. I hardly responded to Prozac and with some symptoms there was a very unwelcome regression. I started to wear surgical gloves on my hands in an attempt to deal with my obsession about AIDS. The pharmacist who sold me the gloves every week, while grateful for the repeat business, must have spent hours trying to come up with an explanation for this unemployed 19-year-old who seemed to need more surgical gloves than a successful surgeon. My fellow learners at a typing course I reluctantly attended must have been equally baffled by the sight of a glove-wearing male youth equipping himself with secretarial skills. They probably thought, "That's going to go down well in the first interview."

After a couple of months, I no longer thought that I was stepping on babies. This feature of the illness disappeared as inexplicably as it had arrived. I drove as little as I could and my existence became progressively more circumscribed. After fighting OCD for so long, I was relieved to be given permission to spend time at home by people who knew I was ill. This relief was the only thing that enabled me to tolerate the phenomenal boredom. I was so shell-shocked from my experiences with OCD that I preferred this nothing existence to trying to cope in the real world.

What changed in 1995 was my personality. The subtle shifts in who I was were driven by a lack of confidence. I remember being at a braai (barbeque) and sitting on the periphery holding my mother's hand like a child on the first day at a new school. I see confidence as the knowledge that you can perform and deliver. I had lost that knowledge through years of academic decline and eight months of being ruled by my obsessions. I took private lessons with a view to writing my 'A' level Maths again but I pulled out just before the exam. I tried to combat my difficulties with driving; but I made no headway. These and other failures added to the sense that I could not deliver.

The diagnosis meant increasingly little as time wore on, because the things I feared retained the status of things that I believed could have happened. If I returned home from a particularly bad drive, the knowledge that I had OCD in no way diminished the terror of prison and the hours of going over the journey in my mind. Hundreds of days have been lost over the years to the panic and the ruminations. How do you get excited about the Christmas holidays if you think the police might be looking for you? What is the point of studying for exams if you are going to die of AIDS? This sense of imminent tragedy made a mockery of ambition and my sense of a future. My assertiveness faded with my confidence. I should have stormed into the office of my Zimbabwean psychiatrist in June that year and said:

"What is going on here? I have been on Prozac for months now and I still have every symptom except one. Do these rubber gloves I'm wearing not make you think that your profession's intervention is not working? Is this how my life is going to be? Because if it is, I am not interested. You have no idea how humiliating this is for me. How on earth am I supposed to go back to university next year? Just have the guts to give me a prognosis and let me decide whether I want to continue this farce."

Many psychiatrists and people who meet me now for the first time would say that I have made a lot of progress. As I have noted, I did experience significant and sustained relief from the terrifying aspects of my OCD symptom profile on an elevated dosage of Risperdal. This relief was eight years after diagnosis. But my yardstick for recovery stems from a statement quoted in David Horrobin's *The Madness of Adam and Eve*. A colleague of his said, "In psychiatry the only real measure of recovery is that the patient is paying tax, preferably not at a minimal level." Risperdal has given me enough relief that I can drive a car to work with only minimal OCD but the compulsive checking that I still battle with in formal employment – checking that is similar to that which I experienced at school and university – has had a significant influence on my inability to hold down a job for more than a year. As a result, my CV is so compromised by illness that I stand little chance of any sort of a formal career. I am not a psychiatrist but from where I'm sitting that is an unambiguous failure to recover in terms of the above criterion.

Fly Fishing For Sharks

I started to assume that psychiatry had nothing to offer so I stopped going to see the hapless fellow. There was very little open forum discussion within my family about my condition. My mother remembers being told by the psychiatrist in Johannesburg, "If your son takes this medication, he won't recognise himself in a few weeks."

On occasion I have called my mother 'Mom Quixote' to reflect her buoyant optimism on most matters. The psychiatrist's statement was something that, as a mother, she quite understandably adopted as a prognosis. When it became obvious that his statement was grossly inaccurate, her belief in a rapid and full recovery was altered to the status of a quixotic conviction that my OCD was bound to clear up someday. I implicitly felt something similar about the course of the illness and, with hindsight, this paradigm was a vitally important coping response in the short term.

The weakness of this approach was that hope and optimism began to replace proactive intervention by myself, my support network and my doctors. In defence of my psychiatrist, he was not able to do much if I didn't make any appointments. In defence of hope and optimism, they provided partial compensation for the fact that his hands were tied by the limits of his profession and the deficiencies of modern psychopharmacology.

One of my psychiatrist's suggestions was that I keep an elastic band around my wrist at all times. The idea was that this was to be elongated and released every time I was driven to act on a compulsion. The resultant stinging sensation was meant to have a moderating influence on my compulsive thoughts and behaviour. This was a woefully ineffective means of treatment.

I've got permanent scars on my stomach from trying to stop my compulsions with a more drastic variant of the elastic band intervention. At one point I became so angry with myself for not resisting them that I heated a piece of metal with a cigarette lighter and burnt holes deep into my flesh. It didn't work in the same way that thrusting a red-hot poker up your behind will not stem the flow of a bad case of diarrhoea.

What was next, a course of leeches? Stinging yourself with an elastic band to treat OCD is not medicine, its self-flagellation. The emotional pain of OCD is difficult enough to cope with. Being told to self-medicate with physical pain is irresponsible because many OCD patients are extremely hard on themselves and they will start to think, "If mild pain isn't working, maybe I should really hurt myself." I know this because the scars on my stomach tell me so. In the world of OCD, few things do as much damage as making a patient feel responsible for either his illness or his lack of progress.

As 1995 drew on, we had to start taking some decisions about the road ahead. Although I wanted to return to UCT, it was obvious that a smaller, more manageable university would make more sense. At least to begin with, it needed to be a place where I could walk everywhere because driving was still such an issue. Rhodes University, in South Africa's Eastern Cape Province met all those criteria. It was situated in the bucolic hamlet of Grahamstown and had a very vibrant and safe residence system. I applied to a residence called College House which had only fifty students and a reputation as a cohesive and supportive environment.

I applied to study Economics and Philosophy. Undergraduate Economics at Rhodes entailed - from what I could glean from the prospectus - a very mild quantitative element; and Philosophy didn't appear to be quantitative at all. I felt that these courses would insulate me from the OCD associated with mathematical disciplines such as finance and, to a lesser extent, accountancy. I also felt that I would cross the bridge of compulsive re-reading when I came to it.

As a devoted fan of Monty Python, it was difficult to avoid the conclusion that choosing a career in accountancy was tantamount to heresy. I knew precious little about balance sheets, auditing or accounts receivable but I was taking the Pythons' word for it that this discipline was soporifically dull and to be avoided at all costs. When I applied to Rhodes, I had no idea how much qualified accountants with a career in finance were paid. Nor did I know how comparatively little remuneration - or for that matter, employment opportunities - came the way of people with an undergraduate degree in Economics and Philosophy and a history of mental illness.

I arrived at Rhodes in February 1996, a shadow of my former self. In fact the shadow I was then sporting was considerably larger than the one cast by my former self. I had gained about fourteen kilograms in the previous year when food became the means by which I cheered myself up. Prozac is implicated in weight gain, but I would be dishonest if I claimed that it was the only factor that contributed to my corpulent physique.

I strode into College House armed with a suitcase of fairly unstylish clothes, a newly acquired laptop and a six-month supply of anti-depressants. Embarking on what should have been the most exciting years of my life with a vanity bag of Prozac could be viewed as an ominous beginning, but Prozac had achieved precious little in its first year of beavering away at my faulty synapses, and I saw no reason why it should start causing trouble now.

I'm guessing that most secular universities have some fairly impressive binge drinking statistics but the drinkers amongst the Rhodes student body are not to be trifled with. The

University has a fine academic staff and some top notch faculties, but this in no way detracts from its reputation for bacchanalian intemperance. On Friday nights, students would flock to a large room in the Student's Union Building to drink, dance and, if possible, find a partner for amorous pursuits. Intrepid members from a church called His People would sometimes have a big prayer meeting in a side room just down the passage from the entrance to the Temple of Vice, and offer up prayers for the lost souls in the Temple. Sometimes a few of His People would venture out of their prayer room and attempt to dissuade the revellers from continuing with their dissolute activities. This was a wildly unpopular strategy.

I had been told not to drink while on Prozac, which was an unfortunate proscription for someone residing in College House. Our residence pub was called the Toot and Tiger, and this fine establishment was the unofficial status-allocating mechanism in College. It wasn't just drinking prowess that conferred status. Regular attendance, the ability to entertain and a disregard for other engagements during Toot time were also considered important.

I went into the Toot on the first night of orientation week to be greeted by the disconcerting sight of one of my fellow first years vomiting into the large black dustbin next to him. He checked his watch, while vomiting, and proudly announced the exact time of his purge after he had wiped his mouth. He seemed to be delighted to have achieved this feat at such an early stage in the evening. The odd thing was that he appeared to have planned this for years. He was a Grahamstown local, and was thus privy to the mores and customs of his chosen residence. Witnessing an act of premeditated vomiting, and the approval it elicited amongst the other students, somewhat dampened my resolve to make a public announcement that I was on medication and not allowed to drink.

Fly Fishing For Sharks

Toot and Tiger legends down the years were, more often than not, alpha males who would have fitted right into Marlboro County. A couple of them were there that night when I picked my moment and stood up to speak. Anticipating that I might raise an appropriately reverential toast to the Toot and Tiger, I think that it came as a shock when I said, "Ah, um, excuse me guys, I just wanted to let you know that I am on medication and my doctor says I can't drink."

I imagine most of them thought, "Well then, what the fuck did you apply to this residence for?" I was thinking exactly the same thing.

I spent a lot time crying in my room in orientation week and would listen to the nightly sounds of a good time being had by all at the Union. I resolved to focus on my academic pursuits and to maintain a steely disregard for the inevitable opprobrium from my fellow College Knights. In College, we were known as Knights although some of us succeeded in actually inducing rather than relieving distress in many of the damsels we encountered owing to our limited capacity for chivalry. If you had seen me in those early weeks at Rhodes, it is unlikely that the word Knight would have leapt to mind. I was still worried about AIDS, so communal showers and dining halls were places of anxiety and social withdrawal.

A fellow first year noted at dinner one evening that I didn't shower very often. He might have shut up if I told him that I always checked my knife and fork for blood but this incident was before my decision to become an overconfessor. I wish that my reply to him could have been classified as witty repartee. Shame tends to limit one's pool of apposite comebacks, though, and I probably said something inane like, "Well, in Zimbabwe we were taught to save water because we had lots of droughts." No upward adjustment of status or knightliness on that particular evening.

I spent a fair amount of time during orientation week in the periodicals section of the Rhodes Library. If there was a strategy to avoid meeting women, this was most certainly it. It was also not the stuff that Toot legends were made of. Nonetheless, this secluded haven had a wide variety of current affairs and business magazines; and a selection of foreign and regional newspapers.

I was flipping through one of South Africa's weekly financial publications when I happened across a few pages headed with the words, "Top Jobs for Top People". I scanned the columns of vacancies, eager to assess my employment prospects upon graduation. As a result of naivety as much as anything else, I was surprised to discover that, in South Africa at least, the ticket to an exciting career and a hefty salary was to become a Chartered Accountant. This route seemed almost obligatory if you harboured ambitions to work in investment banking in Johannesburg – Africa's financial hub and the seat of its biggest stock exchange. I had never thought of working in Johannesburg but I reasoned, without any further research, that if accountancy opened doors in Johannesburg, it was also likely to do so in New York.

I realise how ridiculous my investment banking dream was, but my refusal to let it go was linked to the denial that informed the optimistic projections of my post-illness future. This denial postponed the day when I accepted that I would have OCD for life. No-one dreams of becoming a dependent adult and I needed an illusion to get me out of bed each morning. As I write this, I know that I will never work for Goldman Sachs. It is comfortable to think that OCD and work permits were the only constraining factors. It is also wrong. The truth is that a lack of talent was, and always will be, the obstacle I disregarded.

There is no formula for deciding to cut your losses and let go of your dreams. The decision itself is comparatively easy, but actually letting go is part psychological diet and part emotional cold turkey. Few truly succeed in this journey. For a small minority, letting go is viewed as a compromise that they feel acutely, and the resultant disappointment in themselves and the world can colour the rest of their lives. After almost a decade, I did manage to let go of the Wall Street dream, perhaps because I was forced by circumstances to accept its almost delusional tenets.

What I haven't managed to do is fully accept my illness. I know I'm ill, but I still Google the search terms 'new psychiatric drugs', 'OCD' and 'Depression' regularly in the hope that I don't have to die like this. Acceptance is made all the more difficult if your situation has just the slightest chance of being reversible.

Back then, on the day of registration at Rhodes, my banking dream was still alive and instead of Economics and Philosophy I signed up for a Bachelor of Accountancy. In doing so, I raised the quantitative element of my academic programme to a level that would have had Grahamstown psychiatrists buying on credit. It is obvious to me now that this spectacularly poor decision was informed by my obsession with being a banker. What was so different about this obsession was that it was so pleasurable to indulge. Thoughts about Wall Street, stellar salaries and the attendant lifestyle were not distressing or anxiety-provoking.

Anxiety disorder obsessions are entrenched by the patient's compulsive responses because the brain becomes accustomed to the temporary relief they provide. Paradoxical though it may seem, the patient develops a type of dependence on the cycle that begins with painful anxiety, is followed by temporary calm and then repeats itself again and again. The relief is emotionally addictive.

For me, Wall Street became an obsessive fantasy that grew more entrenched as I indulged it with magazines, newspapers and books. Maybe the expression 'obsessive fantasy' is tautological. Perhaps a fantasy is simply an obsession that induces euphoria rather than panic. If it is, I wonder whether my predilection for OCD played a part in the extent to which my fantasy distorted my decision-making. In a brain that was not adequately distinguishing between what it imagined and what my eyes saw, did fantasising about working for Goldman Sachs give this scenario some measure of projected reality – a reality that validated the fantasy? Was this the same cognitive malfunction that made me to look in the rear view mirror and over my shoulder in response to the purely mental image of a mangled cyclist or dead baby? Whatever the answer, the sense of eager anticipation I felt in my first Accounts 101 lecture was perhaps one of history's most misplaced emotions.

Chapter XII

Snapping hymens and rewriting the Bible

University became less of a journey of academic awakening and more a time of personal growth through the characters I met, the experiences I had and the lessons learnt from the mistakes I made. The OCD that had affected my academic life in high school began to exhibit a marginal attenuation by the time I started at Rhodes. I say this because I didn't experience as many problems with reading as I had with Dickens. This might have been a token gift from Prozac. It might also have been that academic OCD was the aspect of my symptom profile that yielded partially to the fact that I knew my behaviour was as a result of illness. Academic OCD was still maddeningly frustrating and my reading speed remained well to the left of the bell curve; but I could sometimes catch myself mid-compulsion and say, "For fuck sakes, Andrew, you know you don't have to do this." This insight had a minimal effect but I think it made the difference between getting a degree and dropping out.

The Bachelor of Accounting was a four-year programme but I didn't last the first year. For me, OCD and Accountancy were mutually exclusive. I tried for a while but I just couldn't see a way through. There is no better way to explain the relationship between me and Accounts than to tell you my mark in the final exam at the end of first year was...a drum roll please...16 per cent. I switched back to Economics and Philosophy in the second year. This was a three-year programme but failed courses, repeated courses and missed prerequisites meant that my stay at Rhodes was extended by a year.

Over the four-year period, I passed 20 courses and failed six. There were some respectable passes in the high 60s and mid 70s but nothing prodigious. In my second year, I wanted to drop out of University and failed all my courses at mid-year on purpose. I was surprised that they didn't ask me to leave but I had written a letter to the Dean of Students when I applied to Rhodes, in which I explained some of the limitations imposed by OCD. This might just have saved me. (It also caught me slightly off guard in the third year, when I received a letter from the administration office asking me if I wanted to compete in the Special Olympics. The University's records had me listed as a student with a disability. I didn't bother to correct the misunderstanding and left them thinking that my prosthetic leg fell off on the way to each of those four exams I failed - or whatever it was that prevented my exclusion from the university on academic grounds.)

Philosophy is an odd subject. With every new subject I have started since my first days at school, I have arrived at the first lesson assuming that I didn't know anything. At university I realised that not everyone adopts a similar position. An irritating minority of my classmates considered themselves Philosophers before they arrived at university. At best, they seemed to have signed up to the course merely to fill in the gaps. At worst, they were desperate to show the rest of us how brilliant they were. I often felt like blurting out, "Sitting cross-legged on the lawn with your alternative friends, smoking weed and attempting to be profound is a tried and tested way of producing meaningless drivel. Now go to the library and read up on the great philosophers before you waste our time questioning everything they said."

I stopped going to lectures for a while because the poor lecturer was continually harassed by these 'philosophers' who felt that Kant, Nietzsche, Wittgenstein, Plato and Descartes had not thought things through sufficiently. In my

Fly Fishing For Sharks

'O' level Physics class. a friend of mine had raised his hand one day to say that he disagreed with Kirchhoff's laws. Our Physics teacher was quick to respond. "Well, Lukas," he said, "in that case you have a lot of textbooks to correct."

I passed Philosophy 3 with 69 per cent by familiarising myself with the writings of the great thinkers, rather than trying to rewrite them. Many 'philosophers' were below me on the results sheet. There was nothing special about my grade but my position above the 'philosophers' was immensely satisfying.

In the early weeks of the first year I held firm to my resolution to focus on academic pursuits. I didn't go out to the Union or frequent the Toot. OCD was in the driver's seat for many of the hours I spent at my desk. It was like being back at school and it came as a huge disappointment to realise that I was facing four years of the same problems. Even with the marginal improvement I referred to earlier, it was in that first term that I lost the joy of acquiring knowledge for the second, and what seemed like the final, time.

I found Economics interesting but I hated re-reading paragraphs and getting stuck turning the pages of a textbook. When I had been diagnosed, I was sent for psychometric testing that included establishing my IQ. I managed to convince the chap administering the test to dispense with protocol and let me know my exact score. I have read enough to know that IQ is a controversial measure of intelligence. Nonetheless, my score was the confidence boost that I really needed at the time after my decline at high school. It was high enough to give me hope that - with the right therapy and medication - I could do well at university and regain some lost self-esteem.

It was on a Wednesday evening about six weeks into the first term when I realised that the anticipated comeback was stillborn. I had decided that, although it was clear that OCD would hinder my studies, I was not going to allow it to let me continue as a bland outsider in the social life of College House. I knew that most of the guys there didn't think much of me and, worse still, that it was my fault.

Wednesday evening was a party night at Rhodes and the contrast between the frustration with my work and the fun of the Toot stirred something within me. I looked long and hard at the door, took one last glance at a sentence I was re-reading, stood up, slammed the book shut and walked downstairs to the Toot.

To the cynical outsider, the Toot was simply a place where rowdy young men got drunk and sang lewd songs at the top of their voices. The harshest critics of this fine establishment were a certain breed of female undergraduate – characterised by a misappropriated feminism that led them to desire tame and androgynous masculinity, or none at all – and, for the first few weeks of term, me. An impulse analogous to the one that drove Alexander the Great and drives corporate empire builders was behind the College Knights' determination to outdo each other in beer consumption. It doesn't matter that history will not record their exploits. Complaining that the outcome is strained livers and drunken excesses is ignoring the underlying mechanism and simply misses the point.

When I arrived at the Toot, I was greeted by a guy called Trevor Pocock. He was in dire need of a visit to the toilet but, in the interests of welcoming an unexpected newcomer, he ignored the frenzied pleadings of his bladder, said that he was glad that I had come and then launched into an impassioned disquisition on the camaraderie, humour and memories that were available to the those who came to the

Fly Fishing For Sharks

Toot. This disquisition was so thorough that Pocock was forced to relieve himself in the Warden's flowerbed.

When I sat down and took the first sip of beer, there were no questions about why I had changed my mind about drinking on medication. Perhaps those gathered had originally thought that I was hiding behind medication, rather than admitting that I didn't want to drink. It is true that doctors discourage heavy drinking on most psychiatric medication but if I had really wanted to get hammered, I would have ignored that advice, as I do now. The first day in the Toot, I had indeed been hiding behind Prozac; but on that evening six weeks later I felt that the deleterious effects of mixing alcohol and fluoxetine hydrochloride – Prozac's chemical name – could not be worse than the tacit opprobrium of my peers in College House. There was no peer pressure involved. I simply wanted identity and a sense of belonging.

Standard operating procedure in the Toot was to binge drink and talk at the top of one's voice. At times, those gathered would break into song. There was the College House War Cry which was an emphatic declaration that we intended to drink a lot and, where possible, have sex. The song made no reference to academic excellence and its subtext was that anyone attempting to foil our plans would be given very short shrift. The other songs would have kept us all celibate if any female students happened to overhear us. At least that is what I thought the first time I heard them.

I envisaged lonely winter evenings for the lot of us the first time I joined a mob of College boys venturing from the Toot to the Students' Union, with a cursory shower in between. This grim prognosis was based on the uninhibited chants of "Show me the front end of your bum," and, worse, "Show me the gap between your legs" that issued forth from College's finest Knights as we made our way to the Union. Not wanting to spoil the party, I did join in but felt strongly that these injunctions formed a questionable strategy considering that, on the way to the Union, we passed a significant number of the very women we intended to woo back to our rooms later that night. Needless to say, no front ends of bums or gaps between the legs were revealed in response to our crude solicitations.

The next morning on my way to breakfast, however, I noticed a number of nervous female undergraduates vacating the College House premises as fast as their high heels would carry them. I concluded that they obviously hadn't stumbled to the Union at the same time we did. I was very proud of the Knights who had succeeded in this regard.

There was a chap in College called Al Grinham who had an infectious enthusiasm for everything. He would say things that many of us would like to have said, if only we had cared less about what other people thought of us. There were some His People in College House who would periodically erect posters detailing their latest campaign to save souls or eradicate sin. A few of these posters were openly antagonistic. I remember one that read, "Get a life, you loser – life everlasting." Thank Zeus that Grinham was not in College when that little gem was displayed. But he was there when a poster appeared on the door of the common room with the words, "Grahamstown for Jesus," written in large bold letters. Grinham happened upon this poster and, with all the derision he could muster, he was heard for miles around to say, "I'M SURE JESUS DOESN'T GIVE A FUCK ABOUT GRAHAMSTOWN."

When Grinham had a hangover, it wasn't just a hangover. He would stagger into the common room and announce that he had been afflicted with "nine cerebral brain tumours." No-one cared about the tautology because Grinham had captured the essence of what we all felt. At the Toot initiation one year, he proclaimed to the first years that he expected "to hear the sound of hymens snapping all over Grahamstown tonight."

For me, the quintessential Grinham comment came one Sunday evening after the traditional eight o'clock movie. The film was about a Vietnam veteran struggling to build a life for himself on his return from the war. He is eventually killed in a mining accident. All of us were deeply moved. After a long silence following the end of the movie, I said, "Well, I am off to write an anthology of poems." A chap called Mark Rainer said, "I will see your anthology and raise you one." Grinham had the last word and it was nothing to do with a competitive desire to say something more heartfelt than the two of us. He too had been moved by the film and needed us to know the extent of his emotional response. He stood up, walked towards the door and said, "I'm off to rewrite the Bible." If he had done so, I am sure Jesus would have started to give a fuck about Grahamstown.

One of the few true individuals I have ever met lived across the passage from me in College House. Geoff and I met late one evening when he barged into my room, pulled up a chair and began telling me about his evening at the Union. I raised no objection because he was one of the first people to reach out to me in those early weeks. I think he might have seen me opening my door with my elbow and, although he didn't know about OCD, he was intrigued, whereas others would have stayed away. We got to know each other in a series of these well-past-midnight conversations.

Geoff seemed to be immune to the societal pressures and consumerism that straightjackets so many of us. In an attempt to take back some of what OCD has stolen from me, I have recently read and thoroughly enjoyed quite a few of the works of Dickens; and I now think of Geoff as someone Dickens might well have included in one of his books, had he met him. Geoff had a toothbrush whose few remaining bristles were at right angles to those on a regular brush. I asked him how often he changed his toothbrush and he replied, without the slightest hint that perhaps he was unusual, "Oh, about once a year." His teeth looked healthy and his breath was normal, so who was I to suggest amendments to this frugal approach to his dentition. I told him that I changed my toothbrush as soon as the bristles looked unruly. Geoff looked at me as if I was a profligate Saudi Prince.

He was passionate about fishing. I was walking back to College House from lectures one afternoon when I spotted him making his way towards me with his fishing rod, tackle box and an extra spring in his step.

"Geoff, what are you doing? I thought you had your Maths tut this afternoon."
"I do, but it's such a good day for fishing that I've decided not to go."
"Shit, Geoff, I thought you couldn't miss another tut."
"Very true, Stats, but I'm going there now to explain that I can't miss a fishing day like this either."
"Good luck, chum."

As it transpired, Geoff's Maths professor was surprisingly amenable to his student's plans for the afternoon. Most students who miss tutorials would never think of informing their tutor that they intended to do so. Geoff was granted a reprieve on condition that he completed the work in his own time. For many men - including Maths professors - a sincere desire to go fishing is a perfectly acceptable excuse for taking the afternoon off. And so it should be.

You will have noticed that Geoff referred to me as "Stats". This was my nickname at University. It was short for Statistics but had nothing to do with a special aptitude in that discipline. I was sitting quietly in the common room one

Fly Fishing For Sharks

Saturday waiting for lunch. Most of College House was also in the room watching South Africa play Pakistan at cricket. Just before we all left for the dining hall, someone shouted, "What the hell is the population of Pakistan?" A hitherto mum Andrew Alexander said, "It is 133 million." There was a stunned silence. I can only speculate that they were thinking, "What breed of individual from Southern Africa keeps his finger on the pulse of Pakistani demographic data? For that matter, why the hell does he know it down to the last million? He could have said, 'Don't quote me on this, but it is about 130 or 140 million,' couldn't he?"

The reason I didn't is that 133 was the figure that had lodged itself in my head when I was looking through *The World Almanac and Book of Facts,* 1996 edition that my sister had bought for me. I have an odd memory. Without asking my permission, certain bits of information simply find themselves a comfortable chair in a well-lit corner of my mind and make themselves at home. Quotes from Blackadder and Monty Python do a similar thing. I wish I had more of a say in the matter because I could have used a co-operative brain during many an exam. A week or so after the cricket incident, Rob Walter introduced me to his beautiful girlfriend, Monya, as Andrew "Statistics" Alexander. The name stuck and I earned my first mark of identity in College House.

I was lying in bed one evening when I heard Geoff returning home from the Union with what sounded like a girl. I got up to investigate and was instantly stricken with a bad case of envy when I saw who it was that followed him into his room: a potently attractive Jewish girl who always injected a much-needed dose of chic into campus fashion. A number of girls were attracted to Geoff but I don't recall him ever having a long-term relationship during our time at Rhodes. I think his definition of high-maintenance women were those who expected him to visit more than once a month.

About five minutes after they had closed the door, I heard a shrill yelp that seemed to herald an end to the proceedings. There followed some rapid but muffled dialogue, the door opened and I heard the sound of hurried feet making their way along the passage and down the stairs. I opened my door to find Geoff standing in his doorway looking puzzled.

"Geoff, what the hell happened?"
"What a yuppie," was his dismissive reply.
"Why do you say that?"
"I was scaling fish on my bed this afternoon and some of the scales must have ended up on my pillows when I cleared away the newspaper. She lay down and got some of them on her cheek and made a huge fuss about it. What a yuppie."
"Geoff, you don't have to be a yuppie to dislike getting fish scales on your face. Where are the fish now?"
"In my basin."
"Geoff, you are one of a kind, my friend."
"Hey, Stats, do you want some melba toast?"

I declined Geoff's offer because I knew that his melba toast had started life in the dining hall a few weeks previously as perfectly good slices of bread. The crispness of Geoff's stash owed nothing to time well spent in a toaster.

Chapter XIII

The wages of Carlsberg Draft

At the end of 1999, I returned to Zimbabwe having gained a degree and lost my virginity. I have never enjoyed losing anything so much. I can't speak for the wonderful girl who gave two and a half years of her life to be my girlfriend but I found fornication to be a fantastic pastime. With the careful use of birth control pills, we made it through the entire period without starting a family and I have to say that premarital sex amongst consenting adults is the subject of a ridiculous amount of criticism it doesn't deserve. As Sam Harris might say, "If premarital sex is a sin, who is the victim?" In my case, it was my poor girlfriend for the first couple of months until I learnt the rudiments of intercourse.

OCD went on sabbatical for the following six months. I am almost sure that this temporary reprieve had nothing to do with Prozac. If it did, "effective after five years" is hardly something a marketing department would want to splash across a billboard. Life without the illness was right up there with fornication. Having not seen a psychiatrist for four years and now confident that I would never have to see one again, I made an appointment with the family GP. I told him that I was healed and asked him if I could stop taking Prozac. He raised no objections, but did say that the discontinuation must be gradual to avoid withdrawal symptoms. Having never felt remotely high on Prozac, I was somewhat offended that I would pay a price for throwing my remaining pills in the dustbin that very evening.

Three months after my return to Zimbabwe, the country began to unravel with the first wave of farm invasions and the political violence and intimidation that led up to the parliamentary elections in June 2000. I was teaching English at a school in Harare and studying postgraduate Economics via correspondence when the problems started. Initially, I viewed the disturbances as a temporary phenomenon, engineered to garner votes ahead of the elections. I started to panic when the 'war veterans' - as they were inaccurately known - began murdering white farmers. The most unsettling feature of these murders was that organs of the State such as the army and the police were implicated in the crimes. Footage on international news channels showed frenzied mobs looting farmsteads and burning vital infrastructure.

I had attended enough Economics lectures to know that subverting property rights was a very efficient way of destroying an economy. The distortions of the colonial period could not be addressed with more distortions; and nobody learns anything about commercial farming by dispensing with the rules of commerce. Some 85 per cent of the commercial farms in Zimbabwe had been purchased on the open market after independence. In many of these transactions, the Government was given the right of first refusal. With greater political willpower, Robert Mugabe's government could have resettled a considerable portion of the rural poor onto more arable land in the twenty years preceding the land invasions.

Although there was little chance of a team of 'war veterans' invading our suburban home in Harare, I became increasingly convinced that the land invasions and political violence meant that Zimbabwe was unlikely to live up to its promise of becoming the Switzerland of Africa. The squandering of Zimbabwe's inherent potential to achieve this odd distinction was a feature of rueful discussion at dinner parties when I was growing up. I had been skiing in Switzerland in 1992 with my family and, after two weeks of committed comparison, I unearthed only one similarity –

both countries were landlocked. Africa is not a very ambitious basis for comparison and the 'Switzerland of Africa' strikes me as an absurd aspirational analogy. If we wanted to be the Switzerland of Africa in an economic sense, we would have to wait for the day when having a Zimbabwean bank account is a global status symbol. My money is on P'yongyang becoming the 'Paris of Asia.'

I decided to go to London to join many of my friends who had already left Zimbabwe. Although I had no claim to a British passport, I was entitled to apply for a two-year working holiday visa because I lived in a country that was still a member of the British Commonwealth. I discontinued my postgraduate studies, took my last 20 mg tablet of Prozac in late May and left for London in early June.

The upheavals in Zimbabwe had the greatest influence on my decision but I would not have had the confidence to get on the flight to London if I thought OCD had any chance of making a comeback. I was uncomfortable leaving my family in a collapsing country; but I intended to spend two years in London and then emigrate to a First World country where farmers' title deeds meant something. My sister Karin was studying at Harvard but my younger brother and parents remained in Zimbabwe. After I had emigrated, I planned to bring them all over to join me in my new home.

My mother's name is Pauline. She is a highly competent woman and a committed mother. Nothing prepares a mother for having a mentally ill child and I fear that her brief appearances in this book might have given you the wrong impression. She had no idea what was happening to me and I have recorded some of her more emotional reactions as evidence of how even an intelligent, rational adult can be utterly at sea when dealing with a child with psychiatric problems. Like all mothers, she just wanted me to be well and to fulfil my potential. She has always been a proactive problem solver, accustomed to fixing situations. I presented a problem that she could not fix and my illness has been a deeply disconcerting experience for her. Often she has felt helpless but she has never stopped trying to help. Even after my suicide attempts, she put on a brave face and worked the phones looking for new psychiatrists and family therapists; and protecting me from unhelpful advice from charlatans who prey on the vulnerable. Of course she has made mistakes, but they were invariably as a result of a restless search for solutions.

My father's name is Bruce. He is a model of stability, a connoisseur of decorum and the seasoned thermostat of my mother's exuberance. Because of my shame our relationship was affected by that day when I was ten and he spoke to me about the sex games. My diagnosis was devastating to him but we have almost never spoken about the illness candidly. He grew up in a home where frank communication was rare and this made it difficult for him to talk openly about emotional issues. In this regard he is like many men of his generation. However, he never judged me and has never complained about the expense. In 2006 when we went as a family to therapy, he spoke openly about how desperate he was to help me. I was so grateful to hear how he felt and it was a tremendous source of comfort to me. Silence is so often misinterpreted as disapproval but my father's silence about OCD was only because he didn't know what to say for fear of making a bad situation worse.

My sister Karin is a powerful character. She very seldom provokes a neutral reaction in others. She is passionate about Africa and has always wanted to work towards improving conditions on the continent. She won scholarships to international schools, Harvard and then Oxford. She could easily have leveraged her network and educational credentials to secure employment in any number of exciting cities around the world. But she chose to return to Africa and follow her conviction that it is not a lost continent. She can be controversial in her views and anyone who exhibits racism in her presence is likely to be humiliated on the spot. For most of the early years of my OCD, she was in a different country but she was steadfast in communicating with me, sending gifts and finding out how I was doing. It was difficult for her to come to terms with an older brother who went from sparring with her to needing her support. Although younger than me, she has, in recent years, taken on the role of older sister and supportive guardian. She is assisted in this role by her husband Adam, a flamboyant actor and a good friend of mine.

My younger brother Rory, seven years my junior, is fine young man. He is sensible, stable, hard-working and extremely practical. He is a model of discretion, always up and about very early after a night of heavy drinking, while everyone else involved is confined to their beds compounding their misery with self-reproach. He is the type of guy you would want flying your plane through turbulent weather. I introduced him earlier when he offered to sit in the back seat of my car and look out the window to reassure me that I hadn't hit anyone. He was twelve at the time. He has retained this sensitivity and consideration for others into adulthood and is much loved by family and friends.

My first impression of London was that people seemed to be in a permanent rush. My friend Heath met me at the airport and we arrived at his home in Southfields in what must have been record time. Heath had to fetch some sunglasses in Wimbledon and I opted to accompany him in order to get a feel for my new neighbourhood. Our conversation was continually interrupted because I kept falling behind. Heath had evolved since he had come to London and was now able to walk as fast as most people jog. I would periodically break into a compensatory jog to catch up with him but my heavy shoes and baggy corduroys meant that I appeared very unatheletic to passers-by. I coined the phrase, "the Wimbledon shuffle" to describe my attempts to keep up with Heath that day and concluded, rather reluctantly, that my days of moseying along were numbered.

I loved my first month in London. So many of my friends from university and Harare were there and the area in which I was staying was heavily populated with Zimbabweans and South Africans. Heath was an excellent guide - once I had learnt to speed up.

I have always derived immense enjoyment from reading newspapers and the leap in quality and variety from Harare to London was as big as it gets. The *Economist* was always available in Zimbabwe and remains my yardstick; but my first visit to a London newsagent resulted in apoplexy. I felt like a kid again, gripped by an irrational desire to purchase everything the minute I set foot in a toy store. I hurried back to the flat with a bag of newspapers and it was almost midnight before I decided that the arcane *Financial Times* supplement I felt compelled to read was, in fact, a bit beyond me. I accumulated a respectable pile of unread newspapers that was in no way helped by the irresistible bumper editions that came out every Sunday.

My parents had generously given me a thousand pounds to keep me going until I found a job. Within the first week it became clear that London had perfected the art of getting people to part with their money; and that the money I started with would facilitate considerably less 'going' than anticipated - especially if I wasn't firm with myself about newsagents and the bookstores on Charing Cross Road.

London's status as one of the world's financial capitals activated the old delusion that I was suited to a career in investment banking. I emailed my CV to several financial recruitment agencies and, after an agonising two weeks, one of them phoned me to arrange an interview. A very pleasant fellow spent a good hour trying desperately to extract something saleable from my CV. He suggested I do a data inputting test, for which I achieved a miserable score. I came away thinking that I should have gone to a university that offered a Bachelor of Excel Spreadsheets, with majors in Formulas and Macros - whatever the hell those were - or at the very least persevered with Accounting long enough to learn how do to a bank reconciliation.

Perhaps because he had heard about the troubles in Zimbabwe, the chap from the recruitment agency agreed to keep me on his books and let me know if anything came up. I phoned him once a day for the following three weeks until he admitted that he was so sick of hearing my voice that he had achieved the impossible and found me a job. He described it as a "foot in the door" position at a reputable City fund management corporation. I reported for duty the next day in my three piece suit and felt very proud as I strode at London pace down Cheapside in the shadow of St Paul's Cathedral, with all the other bankers. But getting my walking speed up to scratch was not nearly as difficult as mastering the Underground at rush hour.

I had to change trains at Bank station. I remember standing on the platform with more people in suits than I had ever seen in my life. A train came rushing out of the darkness of the tunnel, packed with more uncomfortable people than I imagined could ever exist. I thought to myself, "Oh well, obviously no-one will be climbing aboard this one." My admiration for Londoners ratcheted up a notch as I watched everyone - from powerful broad-shouldered men to deceptively meek women in their late fifties - behave like rugby players in a particularly vicious maul. Rush hour on the London Underground is a contact sport.

After the third train arrived, carrying passengers looking like they were bound for the Gulag, I employed the skills I had acquired as a passable 2nd VX prop in my school days and scrummed my way onboard. I spent the journey examining the dandruff of a tall fellow whose neck was five centimetres from my eyeballs. This was a pleasant fate compared with the short woman who was employing her entire quota of back muscles to avoid wedging her hooked and flaring proboscis into my now pungent armpit. I wanted to shout, "Where the hell is the referee?"

I arrived at my place of work and presented myself at the reception desk, where I quoted the name of the person who would be my direct superior. I became a little alarmed when the receptionist said, "Let me take you down to him." Down. Why Down? Miners and sewerage maintenance workers go down to work. Admittedly, the hard science of interior design had made great leaps in the late twentieth century, but I still thought it unlikely that fund managers would want to go about their business in subterranean shafts even if the décor was "to die for". As I followed her down stairways and through corridors, the surroundings became progressively less like the well-appointed office environment I had envisaged.

Dimly lit though it was, the last corridor provided enough light for me to read the words "Mail Room" on the door at the end. In using the expression "foot in the door," the recruitment consultant had certainly journeyed to the twilight zone of semantics beyond which euphemism becomes fabrication. I have read the corporate fairytales in which the hero rises from the mail room to the CEO's office; but as I crossed the hallowed threshold into Stampland, all I could think of was how few women would sleep with Postman Pat.

Fly Fishing For Sharks

I was confident that seventeen years of schooling would have prepared me for the intellectual rigours of sorting letters. If not, I still had the two years at nursery school to fall back on which, come to think of it, was all I really needed. This confidence was the only positive emotion I could muster that morning because when that far down, the bottom rung of the corporate ladder was reachable only by hot air balloon.

During the day it transpired that the fund managers only needed me to sort mail for that Monday. This elicited mixed emotions because although I hadn't had one of my most stimulating days, I was in dire need of a job. I received a call from my friendly recruitment agent and was on the verge of having a few stern words with him when he said, "Good news, Andrew, there is a position open in the cash management department. They need a temp for nine months. All the paperwork has been done in preparation for today, so I suggested they take you. They agreed, and you've got the job." I went home feeling lucky.

The trouble began on the first day in cash management. My job was very simple. I was issued with a pile of cheques written by people whose money was managed by the company. Using this information, I then accessed their accounts on a computer and effected the necessary changes. OCD made its unwelcome comeback with the very first cheque.

Account numbers and banking codes meant that I was entering long strings of digits in order to access the account details. The overwhelming obsession was that I was making mistake after mistake. I was gripped by a pervasive sense of myself as omni-fallible. The need for accuracy and the checking involved was reminiscent of my 'A' level Maths exam. The checking intensified under the additional burden of knowing that I was being paid to process these cheques.

This provided OCD with a new lease on life. I was deeply concerned about getting into trouble or being fired for incorrectly altering a client's balance. The appropriate response would have been vigilance but I began heading rapidly for paralysis.

The office was air conditioned to a very pleasant temperature but beads of sweat ran down my back as the day wore on. The pile of cheques needed to be processed by 4 o'clock each day. As this time approached, I realised that I had a very slim chance of completing the work. I attempted to speed up but this aggravated the OCD, as it had always done. The head of cash management had been watching my progress and stepped in at about 3 o'clock to assist me. I watched in amazement as she processed the remaining three quarters of the cheques in about half an hour.

Familiarity with the task and advanced keyboard skills were contributing factors to her alacrity; but having a sense of perspective about the scope for inaccuracy and, more importantly, an appropriate conception of mistakes as reversible must also have boosted her productivity. Unfortunately for sufferers, OCD is distinguished by its almost complete lack of perspective. This provides a fertile breeding ground for inappropriate conceptions. She didn't seem impressed with my first day of managing cash. And neither was I.

The following three days were no better. If anything, I became slower. At the end of each day there was a pile of unprocessed cheques and someone had to be drafted in to complete the work. It came as no surprise when I was fired at lunch time on the fourth day. The head of cash management was perceptive enough to realise that I had a problem of some sort. Her desk was directly behind me and she must have seen me repeatedly tracing my entries on the computer with my index finger. The number of times I picked up processed cheques and held them up to the screen to confirm my entries was also unlikely to have escaped her notice. But she could see that I desperately needed work and, in an unsolicited act of kindness, offered to keep me on in the department and find odd jobs for me to do.

The return of OCD and the dismal performance in my first real job were responsible for a rapid lowering of my self-esteem. On the Monday of that week, I had entered the mail room feeling mightily aggrieved that someone such as me should end up in a place like that. By Friday I was starting to think that my strengths might lie in filing and photocopying. I was also shocked by how quickly OCD had become a significant part of my life again. I suppose I should have foreseen that the OCD linked to my academic life would have caused problems in a job requiring accurate clerical work to be performed quickly.

In hindsight, the clean bill of health I had given myself six months previously had applied only to the symptoms related to AIDS, babies and driving; and I had naively assumed that the academic OCD would follow suit. In all my time at school and university, I had never been under the kind of time pressure I experienced with those cursed cheques. It proved to be the perfect change in weather for OCD to come out of hibernation.

My second naïve assumption was that OCD's more terrifying manifestations would not also begin to stir from their slumbers. Some of the guys from cash management spent their lunch hour on a Friday at a pub down the road. They invited me along and although I had little to celebrate, I was in need of the anxiolytic effects of alcohol. I was also pining for nicotine which had been a friend in need on many occasions since I began smoking at University. A friend had told me how smoking helped him to concentrate while studying and, after unearthing some scientific evidence to support this claim, I decided to augment my study programme with cigarettes. Initially I smoked only during exams but as time wore on, I found it to be a useful adjunct to my medication.

I returned to the office in a mild state of inebriation and awaited instructions on what I anticipated to be a manageable filing assignment. I was sitting at my desk staring absentmindedly into the blank computer screen when my alcohol-induced tranquillity was obliterated by a series of horrific images. They depicted a horrible car crash that had resulted from my carelessness when crossing the busy road on my return from the pub. Some of the images were like those in Hollywood action films. I saw a car forced into the air as it collided with another one. The car flew off to one side, killing a large number of pedestrians on the busy pavement.

The images were as vivid and terrifying as those that caused me to drive back to my brother's junior school to look for the bodies of dead children in 1994. Panic set in. You would think that six years of living with this type of OCD would have given me some ammunition with which to counteract the onslaught or, at the very least, a heightened level of insight with which to moderate the anxiety. That day in London, though, it was as if I had never been diagnosed.

There were two new elements involved with this episode. First, the obsession was based on an entirely new scenario, albeit with an underlying commonality with earlier obsessions in that it involved people dying as a result of my mistakes. The second element was alcohol and its role was more destructive. As I was compulsively retracing my steps from the pub to the office, the extent to which I doubted the veracity of my recall was intensified by the knowledge that I was slightly drunk. My inner voice was continually using this against me; and as the doubt grew, so did the guilt. OCD

Fly Fishing For Sharks

had put my guilt to good use in the past and this time was no different.

Psychiatrists use the term "aggressive obsessions" for those obsessions that involve the fear of having caused harm to others. The return of these aggressive obsessions to my symptom profile meant that another meltdown could not be ruled out.

About a week later, I went to have a drink with some of my Zimbabwean friends in a pub in Fulham Broadway. I was staying with Sam Carter at the time in Peckham and the journey home involved a combination of underground and overland trains. I arrived at the pub feeling the need for some form of release; drank far too much and left with very little time to spare. I needed to make it to London Bridge at a certain time in order to catch the last overland train home.

At times I had to sprint during the journey home and I was doing all I could to keep the aggressive obsessions under control. My fondness for Carlsberg draft meant that my ability to recall the exact details of the journey was compromised to a greater degree than it had been on the previous Friday at work. As a result, the obsessions that emerged over the following few days were the most intractable in the history of my illness.

The list is as bizarre as it is varied. Amongst others, the imagined crimes included knocking someone down the stairs in the Underground; stabbing someone with the spike of my umbrella as I ran along the platform; causing a bus to overturn on the road outside the pub; and pushing a little girl into the path of an oncoming train. So powerful were these images and so futile were my attempts to reconstruct the journey, that I began to disintegrate rapidly. In addition, the obsessions had gone beyond the point when a physical retracing of the journey would have provided any relief. An intervention of this kind merely entrenches the illness but, if it is not available, the lifespan of any obsession is excruciatingly extended.

Delayed-onset obsessions always bought my life to a halt because as long as they were tormenting me, I faced the prospect that I might have killed people. While this dominated my conscious mind, I experienced immense difficulty getting on with life. A delayed-onset obsession had occurred a few years earlier on my return to university in 1996 after the winter holidays. It happened two weeks after the "event" and became so all-consuming that I spent a considerable portion of the first three weeks of that semester in my room, engaged in compulsive reconstruction of the drive in question.

Life in London quickly became unmanageable. I phoned home during my lunch hour about two weeks after that night out in Fulham. My mother answered the phone and all I could say was, "Mom, it's come back. Everything has come back." She offered to fly to London and help me get through what she assumed to be a temporary rough patch but I was adamant that I needed to come home. I was so desperate that I gave almost no consideration to Zimbabwe's own steep decline.

I spent the rest of the lunch hour at the farewell party of one of the women who worked in cash management. The relief I felt after having taken the decision to return home lifted the lid on a range of emotions that I had suppressed in order to get through each day and I spent a considerable portion of that lunch hour in tears. My colleagues must have thought it odd that I felt so strongly about a departing employee whom I had known for only a few weeks and with whom I had not exchanged a single word. Perhaps they thought I was in love with her. By that stage, I had lost the ability to care.

Fly Fishing For Sharks

Sam and Catrin were very concerned about my return to Zimbabwe. Catrin quite rightly pointed out that it was in political and economic disarray and - more to the point - I was unlikely to receive the quality of treatment that was available in England. She had booked an appointment for me at a Psychiatric Hospital, having researched OCD on the internet. It was quite clear that I should not have discontinued my medication. There was also evidence to suggest that if SSRIs such as Prozac were not effective, other drugs were available and worth trying. It is a source of considerable regret that I didn't listen to Catrin and go to that appointment; but I was frightened and overwhelmed, my mind surging with such horrible thoughts that I wanted to leave London as soon as possible.

A few days before my departure, Sam found me crying and he realised that what was going on inside my head was beyond my ability to cope. Like a father as well as a friend, he walked over and hugged me. I put my arms around him and my tears grew to agonised sobs. I cried aloud, "It's so hard, it's so fucking hard," and he answered, "I know, I know, but you will get through this." To have someone validate what I was feeling, as Sam did that afternoon, gave me a temporary sense of safety and reassurance. The rain stopped and the wind died down as the eye of that particular psychiatric storm passed overhead for the next couple of hours.

Early the following week, Heath and an old junior school friend of mine, Simon Ward, took the afternoon off in order to take me to the airport. I remain extremely grateful to them both because I would have struggled on my own. We were sitting in a café waiting for my boarding call when Simon asked, "So Andrew, what's your plan?" I responded, "This was it."

For old time's sake, I bought a copy of the *Financial Times* to read on the flight. The headline of one article read, "Mugabe government to take 3,000 farms." Considering that there were only 4,500 commercial farms to begin with this was a discouraging turn of events on the eve of my return to Zimbabwe. It was a stark reminder that the sole motivation for my return was to seek refuge at home.

Fly Fishing For Sharks

Chapter XIV

The Komodo bite

My return to Zimbabwe in 2000 saw no diminution in the aggressive obsessions. The OCD associated with driving returned with renewed intensity. I found that I could not shake the obsessions that had arisen in London. I spent a lot of time reconstructing both the journey that had led to OCD's resurgence and the one that eventually led to my departure.

The mental reconstruction of these two journeys and thousands of drives over the years follows a distinct pattern. The goal is to eliminate anxiety from the memory. I consider this to have been achieved when the whole journey or drive is retraced without any anxiety-provoking thoughts. Almost all of an obsession's power to control behaviour is linked to the evolutionary imperative to respond to severe anxiety. If this can be minimised, the obsession becomes much less terrifying.

Take the journey back to Sam's house in Peckham, for example. The reconstruction begins outside the pub. The images in my mind arose from my doubts about whether I had checked the oncoming traffic before crossing the road. The feared result was that a bus had been forced to swerve to avoid me, thus overturning and causing injury and death. The reconstructive process involves imagining myself stopping at the side of the road, assessing the traffic and proceeding across the street without incident, using as much recalled sensory data as I can muster in confirmation of this 'safe' scenario.

The catch is that this new scenario must be uninterrupted by a disturbing thought. If an overturning bus invades the reconstruction, the process has to start again. Again, guilt associated with drinking made it vastly more difficult to counter invasive thoughts. Guilt's leverage was provided by the increased levels of doubt associated with any recall of the journey, as well as an inner voice that implied that because of my inebriation I deserved a horrible fate.

Once a section of the journey has been 'cleared' of the imagined incident, the reconstructive process can move on to the next 'incident'. Depending on the severity of the obsessions and the associated anxiety, the timeframe for reconstructive ruminations ranges from a couple of minutes to a couple of months – as was the case in reconstructing the Peckham journey.

In the Indonesian archipelago there are some islands known collectively as the Komodo Islands, the home of the eponymous Komodo dragons. These are a species of monitor lizard which grow to be extremely large. They have a particularly insidious way of hunting their prey, which include buffalo. In a biological sense, the Komodo dragon is a particularly foul-mouthed creature. Its mouth is so heavily populated with bacteria that one bite inflicts a wound that eventually proves fatal to the quarry.

The poor buffalo or other victim spends the week or so after the bite desperately looking for relief until the infection from the original wound overwhelms its entire body and it dies. This period of dying is the very opposite of going quietly in your sleep, if the *National Geographic* footage I saw was anything to go by. Komodo dragons then gather around and eat the corpse. I imagine that nature has arranged it such that Komodo dragons select only old or dying animals but given the choice of a range of predators, it strikes me that a world-weary buffalo might alter his will to ensure that he was taken out by a team of lionesses rather than the neighbourhood Komodo.

My experiences in the second month in London were my Komodo bite. They were also proof that First World countries like England or Sweden were not easier places in which to be ill, as I had imagined in my counterfactual speculations. Earlier in my story I thought race might be an aggravating psychosocial factor of the OCD I experienced in Zimbabwe. In London, most of the 'victims' in my aggressive obsessions were white people; and, if anything, the obsessions were more powerful. Spending time in prison frightened me equally in Harare, Cape Town or London. It was clear now that OCD would follow me everywhere and find all the aggravating factors it needed.

The effect of the Komodo bite was a progressive weakening of my emotional immune system. This was the infection that was to spread over the following years and culminate in my decision to end my life. The infection manifested as a growing belief that I couldn't cope with life. In fact, it was more than a belief: I became certain that I couldn't cope with life and I had a catalogue of academic and job-related failures to bolster my case. This sense of inadequacy was implicated in and exacerbated by clinical Depression, a symbiotic partnership that proved very difficult to counteract.

One of the things you often hear depressed people say is, "I couldn't get out of bed in the morning." Statements like these are just metaphors, used in the absence of symptoms that are simple to describe. A literal interpretation will lead some people to criticise the depressed as weak willed and emotionally fragile. If they are, it is because of the depression and like ill people everywhere they need love, tenderness and support. Depression is a mood disorder. Everything about it is emotional.

The underlying dynamics of its neurochemistry and neuropathology are yet to be fully understood but the link between emotions and neurotransmitters is widely accepted. I think that most of us exercise much less control over our moods than we think. I am not referring to specific interventions such as chocolate, full-body massages or illicit drugs. I am talking about willpower. If people dispensed with the illusion that we choose all our emotional states and responses to life events, conditions such as depression would be taken more seriously by the general public. Reducing the role of choice to its rightful place would enable the emotionally stable to feel lucky rather than proud - and the depressed to feel unlucky rather than ashamed.

There was a day in August 2002 when I knew for sure that I was depressed. I knew because it was emotionally painful to be awake. My mood had been falling since May but that morning the oppressive despondency and sourceless sadness made consciousness something from which I was desperate to flee. I hauled myself out of bed and reached into my cupboard for the sleeping pills I had used on a recent bus journey. I had no intention of taking an overdose. I just wanted to go back to sleep to escape my mood.

In January that year, my family had moved from Zimbabwe to Cape Town. We were not refugees but economic migrants whose standard of living was under threat from Zimbabwe's economic decline. I decided to return to Rhodes University to study postgraduate Economics. There was a certain grim tenacity in this decision. In the previous year, six months after my return from London, I had tried the same thing at UCT. The Serbian psychiatrist I mentioned earlier had assured me that I would be fine now that I knew that my OCD was caused by the guilt I felt about the sex games I had choreographed as a child. His confidence was such that I left for UCT without any medication. Although Prozac's effect had been minimal, OCD responds well to stress and change and I should have been taking something.

There is an outside chance that the Serbian's theory was correct. It certainly sounded plausible. Unfortunately, it didn't stand up to much scrutiny. No doubt my past influenced the course of my OCD but any insight that I had gained into putative causes of the illness turned out to be of little use. This is not to say that examining causes is unimportant but rather that once activated, the illness needs to be treated with the insights of medicine and not those provided by Freudian psychoanalysis.

My second attempt at UCT was no better than the first. Academic and aggressive obsessions quickly strangled my supply of gritted teeth. The walk from my flat to campus each day yielded a crop of catastrophic maybes about pedestrians I might have pushed into oncoming traffic; or oncoming traffic that I might have caused to veer off the roads that I had to cross at various stages of the journey. Walking around campus added to the backlog of mental reconstructions I had to perform. Lacerating people with knives sticking out of my bag; knocking people down stairs; causing people to get their heads caught in swing doors through which I had passed – OCD's ability to generate new scenarios was proving phenomenal. These hindered my ability to concentrate in lectures and the inevitable unravelling began once again.

I was in constant e-mail contact with the Serbian back in Zimbabwe. I made it very clear to him that I was regressing at an astonishing rate. This spurred him on to increasingly odd motivational metaphors. I remember deriving no comfort from his suggestion that I had parachuted into a pool of shit and, unpleasant though this might have been, I must clean myself off and jump again. Instructions on how to avoid the same pool of excrement on the second jump were not forthcoming. I withdrew from the course a few weeks later and returned home – again. Back in Zimbabwe, I arranged to have coffee with the Serbian. I sat for an hour at the coffee shop waiting for him but he didn't arrive. I never heard from him again.

I spent a lot of time that March of 2001 sitting in our lounge in Harare, smoking cigarettes, drinking coffee and looking out across our lawn which was a verdant green at the end of the rainy season. I plucked up the courage one day to walk to the video store. I didn't want to drive because I was too frightened by what that would entail at a time when OCD was as bad as ever. The walk was about a seven-kilometre round trip and I knew that crossing roads on foot and encountering other pedestrians would test my fortitude. The trip was difficult and I considered turning back a few times but when I arrived home with two videos to watch, I felt proud of myself. It was a small step but when your life becomes unmanageable, any act of defiance against an illness that is rendering it such is a victory that needs to be celebrated - even if only by yourself.

In April, my family planned to go to Cape Town on holiday. I was very reluctant to accompany them because the trauma associated with my second attempt to study at UCT was still a fresh and uncomfortable memory. In addition, I knew OCD would give me trouble in the public places we were bound to visit. I also had no desire to see all the people we knew in Cape Town and have to explain to them what had gone wrong. But I changed my mind and it proved to be a very important decision.

During the holiday we were invited to dinner at the Hulleys'. It was Jane Hulley who had helped me so much in 1995 when I realised that I needed to withdraw from UCT. During the meal, she noticed how withdrawn and listless I was. After telling my mother, "That is just not the Andrew I used to know," she gave her the number of a reputable psychiatrist in Cape Town.

The psychiatrist was an avuncular fellow who listened intently as I told my story. He was of the opinion that the Serbian was guilty of malpractice and therefore someone who could have been sued in a normal country. Based on my limited response to Prozac, he prescribed a drug called Anafranil and a course of Cognitive Behaviour Therapy (CBT). He suggested that I wait until the drug had moderated my symptoms before I started the CBT, because he felt that I wasn't ready to tackle them at that stage.

My parents were with me at the appointment and had we been members of a remote Amazonian tribe, we would have all stood up and done a relief dance. Either that or we would have offered up the Serbian as a burnt offering the moment we returned to Zimbabwe.

The entire treatment process was going to take a few months which meant that someone would have to remain with me in Cape Town at the end of the holiday. Without hesitation, my mother committed to remaining behind and to assuming the role of a co-therapist. Friends of the family rallied around and helped out where they could. Someone lent us a car and another offered us a flat by the sea at a drastically reduced rent.

It was a special time for my mother and me. We had a great deal of time together and her presence at all the appointments and therapy sessions gave her insight into the bizarre condition that had blown her son so far off course. I did respond to the Anafranil, although residual symptoms persisted. OCD's ability to ruin lives is linked to the frequency and intensity of the symptoms. In this regard it is like most illnesses. The severity of an illness is also measured by the extent to which it affects the patient's ability to function at home, at work or interpersonally.

During the hard times, OCD is my fulltime job. An unprocessed obsession will be the first thing I think of when I awake. More will pile up during the day and I will fall asleep in the middle of a reconstructive rumination. Anafranil altered OCD's status in my life from the dominating force to a more manageable factor: it reduced the frequency and intensity of the aggressive obsessions. The terrifying images were no longer associated with such crippling panic and, with the help of CBT, I was able to reduce the associated reconstructive ruminations. Despite the residual symptoms, Anafranil's ameliorative effect restored some of the dignity I had lost as OCD's slave.

True relief from aggressive obsessions took place after the introduction of the antipsychotic Risperdal to my medication regime. As I noted earlier, I hesitate to ascribe an unmitigated causative role to Risperdal because suicide became an acceptable option to me during its therapeutic trial period. I simply don't know what role it played but I do think that admitting suicide into the realm of my coping responses was a significant step.

I was on Anafranil when I started postgraduate Economics at Rhodes in February 2002. Looking back now to the first six months of the course, I wonder what produced my first experience of Major Depression. I didn't have a car and thus had very little OCD to contend with. I had joined the Running Club and this provided me with a close circle of friends. My academic life was progressing well. I even took the step of registering for a course in Mathematical Economics in an attempt to face some of the demons of my academic OCD and I passed comfortably.

Fly Fishing For Sharks

My Maths professor was an eccentric gem of a fellow. His distinctive gait made it look as though he had adult-onset rickets. His bow-legged progress towards the lecture hall was always embellished with a continual redirection of his gaze, probably linked to his remarkable disinclination towards any sort of eye contact. During lectures he would take pains to avoid looking at his students and instead address all manner of inanimate objects in a form of mathematical soliloquy. These were like verbalised internal monologues complete with little chuckles, raisings of the eyebrows and the odd rhetorical gesticulation. He applied his profession's rigorous need for proof to even the most ordinary of statements.

On the last day of term before the April holiday, attendance at his class was very small He turned to the three or four of us in the classroom and, in his strained Polish accent said, "Why so few students?" We told him that most of campus had gone on holiday a day or two early. He thought for a moment or two and replied, "Ah, it's possible." It was as if our statement was merely a hypothesis and he was going to treat it as such until further confirmatory evidence could be gathered. I love eccentrics and this guy was the genuine article.

Anafranil was having some annoying side effects. The first was that my salivary glands went on strike at crucial moments. At all other times, my mouth would have less saliva than a normal mouth but this could be alleviated by the assiduous sucking of sweets. The poor performance of my salivary glands was in stark contrast to the way in which my sweat glands responded to the drug. Above a certain temperature, I literally began to leak.

But these were minor irritants compared with the grand malfunction that took place one evening that February. One of my fellow classmates and I had been exchanging glances on a regular basis. Having been single for almost four years, I required a slightly neurotic tally of sustained glances before I could dismiss the nagging thought that I was the victim of an elaborate hoax.

A good friend of mine called Simon Mapham told me once that picking up women is a numbers game. Even with the help of liquor and the favourable lighting of bars and nightclubs, the single digits in this game of numbers have, in my experience, almost always been very trying and full of errors. These experiences conspired to fuel my suspicions about a situation that, otherwise, had all the hallmarks of the elusive 'first strike' scenario favoured by Cold War military strategists and numbers game champions.

After a few brief conversations, I cordially invited my classmate to visit me at my flat that Friday evening. I felt very encouraged that she accepted immediately because any hesitation might have occasioned a bout of such heavy sweating that her indecision would have turned rapidly to refusal. Friday's sunset heralded a cool evening as I busied myself making my room presentable. I was grateful for the favourable weather but troubled by the realisation that my room might look poorly furnished and uninviting. I decided that this was only a problem until such time as I turned the lights off, having established beyond a shadow of a doubt that the only piece of furniture that mattered for the remainder of the evening was the bed.

Turning the lights off was only the beginning of my problems. I was very attracted to my guest and not at all nervous. As I began to kiss her, my mouth went dry. It wasn't as dire as the time during a job interview when my lips and cheeks stuck to my gums and I lost the power of speech; but it was a dryness that was fiercely at odds with the evening's proceedings. Saliva is the unsung hero of foreplay and I had none of it. We continued to kiss but I knew that if I wasn't enjoying it, she must've been stacking up excuses for a sudden exit. I opted for a change in tactics and began to kiss her in alternative erogenous zones while gently removing her clothes. She began to help me take off mine and I viewed this reciprocity as evidence that disaster had been averted.

Perhaps because of the diversion of the saliva hiccup, it was not until an erect penis was required that I realised I didn't have one. If it had been at least semi-erect, we both would have had something to work with but it was dictionary definition flaccid. There was no going forward from there. I offered an incoherent explanation that included the words 'psychiatric condition' and 'medication', which only served to expedite my guest's search for her clothing. I walked her to her car and bade her farewell. Any glances exchanged in the following weeks were awkward ones.

I can't be certain that the medication was implicated in my impotence but the dry mouth is an acknowledged side effect of Anafranil and the trouble started with that. I felt embarrassed, inadequate and angry that it had happened when I was still so young. I asked my psychiatrist if I could change from Anafranil to another medication.

I wasn't impotent two years later when I slept with a prostitute. Many factors influenced my decision to do that but I can't be certain that my experience with impotence wasn't implicated. My return to potency might simply have been because I had forked out most of my hard-earned Christmas bonus for Delilah's services and was therefore in no mood for backchat from my well-rested penis. Delilah's bosom looked promising until she removed her bra to reveal two things that looked like products of a sausage machine that had run out of meat. I had seen healthier breasts on skeletal famine victims. I thought to myself, "Delilah, for God's sake, you work in the sex industry: what the hell are those things on your chest? My willy is now getting smaller. I wonder if they offer refunds?" After the initial shock, my penis pulled through and Delilah spent the entire proceedings pretending to enjoy herself. She intermittently praised my performance with trite compliments that were about as convincing as a reading on the Geiger counter owned by Chernobyl's most unscrupulous real estate agent of 1987.

Considering that a fear of contracting AIDS had played such a large part in my life, it must seem odd that I went with a prostitute. By that stage, I was taking anti-psychotics which dealt with AIDS-related and aggressive obsessions in a remarkably effective way. I, too, was surprised that, despite the condom, I didn't panic about infection and cancel the transaction; because the OCD that I knew would have insisted on a full body condom that had been triple tested for leaks. I think that another reason for my lack of concern was a belief that I didn't really have a future to preserve. My life no longer seemed precious.

The decline towards the day in August 2002 when I took sleeping pills to escape my mood had begun on the last day of April that year. I was running the longest distance I had ever attempted that day. It was a sixty-kilometre ultra marathon that started in the seaside town of Port Alfred and ended at a school on a hill above Grahamstown. I had trained harder for that run than I had for anything in my life and had been looking forward to testing my body and - more importantly, my mind - on a route that contained some challenging uphill sections. Many of my new friends from the running club were participating in the event and we were all looking forward to a well-deserved celebration the evening after the race.

It was about 4.30 in the morning when the Rhodes contingent drove down to Port Alfred for the start of the marathon. Although it was autumn, the air was warm and dry. At that time of the morning it was still dark and I was looking out into the night, thinking about the race and hoping that the salt tablets I had brought along would prevent the cramps that had caused me so much difficulty in a marathon about a month previously.

What happened on that journey was by no means traumatic like my early experiences with aggressive obsessions but it was unexpected. I began to think that there was no point in running the race. This was odd because I didn't doubt that I could run the distance; or that I would feel a sense of achievement when I completed it. I simply could no longer see how running the race would serve any purpose. A mild sadness followed this change in perspective about the day's events. It was the beginning of a pervasive shift in perspective and mood that led to Depression.

Chapter XV

Sarah's future, Harold's past

The *Diagnostic and Statistical Manual of Mental Disorders* is the textbook that many mental health professionals use to diagnose patients. The most recent edition is the *DSM-IV*. To understand clinical Depression, it is important to extract it from the colloquial realm by using medical terms for emotional states and the *DSM-IV* gives a full list of these terms.

The alternative is, of course, metaphor. Metaphor is an essential tool of the writer, the poet and the singer but it could blur the line between the clinical and the colloquial. The risk of blurring the distinction is already high with depression given its spectrum of varying severity and the number of purely emotional elements in its symptom profile. To illustrate the pitfalls of metaphor, consider the following scenario.

"Doctor, I think I am suffering from depression."
"Andrew, I'm sorry to hear that. There is a checklist that we must go through to establish whether or not that is the case. Please answer the following questions as accurately as you can."
"OK, doctor, that's fine by me."
"Would you say that a dark cloud has settled over your life?"
"I suppose so."
"Would you agree with *Hamlet* when he said, 'How weary, stale, flat, and unprofitable seem to me all the uses of this world!'?"
"Probably."

"On a scale of 1 to 10, please rate the relevance of the expression, 'permanent winter', to your current state of mind."

"Um….about 7."

"Do you yearn for the oblivion and uninterrupted sleep of death?"

"Sometimes."

"Imagine, if you will, a dark and frigid abyss that is four kilometres deep. Metaphorically speaking, how far into the abyss have you descended?"

"If I had to hazard a guess, doctor, I would say about three kilometres."

"Andrew, it seems that you are indeed depressed and, as such, I will write you a prescription for some mood enhancers. Please keep a chart of your progress out of the abyss, assessing your altitude gain as accurately as possible every Monday and I will see you in a month."

According to the *DSM-IV*, the symptoms of depression are as follows:

- Persistent sadness or despair
- Insomnia or hypersomnia in atypical depression
- Decreased appetite or the reverse in atypical depression
- Psychomotor retardation or agitation (essentially, the depressed person becomes either physically sluggish or restless to the extent that a third party would notice the change)
- Anhedonia (this is the term for an inability to experience pleasure)
- Irritability
- Apathy, poor motivation, social withdrawal
- Hopelessness
- A sense of worthlessness, feelings of helplessness, inappropriate guilt
- Suicidal ideation (this refers to thoughts about killing yourself, and is to be distinguished from the act

itself. The danger is that thoughts can become intentions, and intentions can lead to action.)

This list is not exactly what appears in the *DSM-IV*. I got it from my trusty *Time* almanac, whose authors got it from a report on mental health by America's Surgeon-General. I cross-referenced the *DSM-IV* on the internet, made some amendments to my list and am now obsessing about how to deal with the gnawing sense that the list is compromised and I must start again. But I have decided to leave it as it is. OCD and a few psychiatrists might grumble about certain aspects of the list but Depression would recognise itself without any difficulty. That is all that matters at the moment.

You don't have to exhibit all these symptoms to be diagnosed with Depression but it certainly helps if you do. I had atypical Depression and therefore I overslept, consumed abnormal amounts of food and became very sluggish. I was never very irritable but otherwise I experienced all the other symptoms to a fairly severe degree. Lack of energy, poor motivation and a pervasive sadness were, of course, disabling. They were also maladaptive in a world that requires roughly the opposite. I reluctantly ruled out a career in sales at the time. The most debilitating aspect of my experiences with depression was - and continues to be - a sense of crippling helplessness.

Earlier in my story, I referred to the book *Why Zebras Don't Get Ulcers* by Robert M. Sapolsky, who suggests that the serotonin theory of depression is more complex than originally thought. Later in the book, I came across a concept that seemed to link my OCD experiences to the eventual development of Depression. Professor Sapolsky describes a study in which a rat was put in a cage, the floor of which was constructed so that the entire floor was electrified. The poor rat would receive a shock wherever he went. The shocks weren't fatal but they weren't ticklish either. Predictably enough, once the cage floor was activated, the rat had a terrible time as he scrambled around trying to find a section of floor that didn't hurt. Later in the study, the rat was transferred to a cage in which only certain sections of the floor were electrified. The expectation was that he would explore his new surroundings, and establish for himself which parts of the cage were safe and which were to be avoided.

What happened instead was that rat became passive, curled up in a corner of the cage and stayed there. It was from this study, and others like it, that the concept of 'learned helplessness' was developed. The theory is that if an animal - or a human - is exposed to a highly stressful or dangerous situation in which its 'fight or flight' response is blocked or ineffective; and if this situation persists for long enough, it will eventually learn that it is helpless.

In nature, an ineffective 'fight or flight' response usually results in death. Hence, very few zebras are found curled up on the plains of Africa feeling debilitated by learned helplessness. For a start, they would soon be eaten and forget all about it. Learned helplessness arises from the repeated experience of traumatic situations that involve a sufficient threat – imagined, in the case of OCD – to activate the panic mechanism. These situations might involve the threat of death but the important thing is that they are traumatic; that the organism's response to the threat is ineffective and that they happen again and again until the organism gives up trying. In the first cage, the rat could neither attack nor flee from the electricity; then, when he was transferred to the second cage he applied the lessons of his helplessness. When there is nothing you can do, do nothing. As Sapolsky notes, when an organism stops mounting coping responses, it is really in trouble.

Many of my experiences with OCD involved a situation in which my 'fight or flight' response was compromised and - in some cases - futile. Obsessions would activate my 'fight or flight' panic response and compulsive actions or thoughts were employed against the imagined threat. The first compulsive fight response was very often ineffective, resulting in repetitive compulsions. Because my panic mechanism was activated by my mind and not an external threat, a flight response was similarly ineffective.

My brain was the dangerous animal that my body was designed to flee from. If the Obsessive-Compulsive cycle became too crippling over time, I withdrew from whatever activity provoked it. Whether it was driving a car or doing Maths homework, walking in public or touching unchecked surfaces, I withdrew from the helplessness of OCD. This withdrawal sounds like a 'flight' response but it is not an instinctive reaction like that of a panicked or threatened organism. It is a learned response. It stems from traumatic memories of actual or perceived helplessness.

My experiences were not a volt-for-volt reflection of the rat's ordeal but they were certainly analogous. I believe that most of the helplessness that I felt when I was depressed was helplessness that OCD had taught me. As I noted earlier, my first experience of Depression occurred during a time when OCD was much less of a factor in my life, and thus its etiology would include a list of other causative factors. In addition, learned helplessness - although the dominant feature of my Depression - was not the only symptom and many of the others were unrelated to OCD.

I have introduced the link between OCD and learned helplessness in attempt to show that OCD influenced the specificities of my experience with Depression in the same way that sexuality and religion influenced the symptom profile of my OCD. Learned helplessness was also the most dangerous aspect of my Depression because, as I mounted fewer and fewer coping responses, the belief that I couldn't cope segued into conviction and in my mind, suicide seemed the only coping response left.

I was new to depression when I took the sleeping pills in August 2002 when I naively assumed that more sleep would remedy the situation. Needless to say, when I opened my eyes around midday, things were no better.

The deterioration in my mood from the morning of the marathon in late April to that morning in August was as inconvenient as it was undeniable. I needed to complete my postgraduate degree in order to bolster my perforated CV; then find myself a job that allowed me to cover costs and whittle away at both the interest and the principal of my student loan. In my world, an episode of Major Depression was the character-building experience I needed least. The onset of this episode was undeniable but the defence mechanism of denial is designed to take the 'un' out of 'undeniable'. I did this by focussing on how inconvenient depression would be at that stage of my life and assuming that it would respond to the anti-depressants I was already taking every night for OCD.

Depression is deceptive because, unlike severe physical pain, it tempts you to continue coping with subtle but temporary, upward fluctuations of mood and a gradual onset of symptoms. These factors give rise to hope and mask a trend line that is leading downwards. The intensity of extreme physical pain usually prompts us to visit a doctor and demand relief. The relative tolerability of the slow onset of depressive symptoms often means we delay intervention until our lives fall apart. Depression is a stealth bomber – and there goes my attempt to avoid metaphor.

Denial wasn't a sustainable response with OCD; and the same applied to depression. When the sleeping pills wore off that day in August 2002, my denial broke and I realised that I needed to find help, as I had done in February 1995 at UCT.

Outside the medical profession, I think Depression is considered one of the world's poorest excuses for sick leave or diminished capacity. People often ask "What have you got to be depressed about?" as a result of conflating the clinical and colloquial uses of the word. Admittedly, depressing life events can increase the risk of depression but the fact that, say, not every bereaved spouse moves from grief to depression suggests that other factors are involved. 'Depression' is a specific medical noun; whereas 'depressing' is an overused adjective and the twain meet only occasionally.

Looking at the list of *DSM-IV* symptoms, it is not difficult to see how the casual observer would view Depression more as a function of attitude and choice, than of illness. I imagine that this approach to Depression informs much of the prejudice and misunderstanding directed at the illness. If I had never experienced depression, I assume that I would also be unsympathetic to sufferers. As I noted earlier, I suspect that all of us have less control of our emotional states than we think but I think that this assertion would be furiously contested by many. Moreover, it could be viewed as self-serving. Perhaps a more nuanced assertion would be that some people are less able to control their emotional states than others and this makes them vulnerable to mood disorders.

Whatever the case may be, I had a sense that phoning someone and telling them I was depressed was unlikely to elicit the same response as informing them that I thought I was stepping on babies or was being infected with AIDS from contaminated cutlery.

I was at a loss as to who to contact but I needed to talk to someone. Grahamstown has a public psychiatric facility that I had often passed while out running and I thought I would go there to find some help. It was about five kilometres from where I lived and for similar reasons to the ones that prevented me from phoning, I didn't ask anyone to drive me to the hospital. So, still slightly drowsy from the sleeping tablets, I set off with a noticeable lack of spring in my step. It was a cold day in late winter; the streets were largely empty and a low grey cloud drained the buildings and vegetation of colour. I wish I was making this up. I wish it had been a summer's day and that I had been intercepted by a passing carnival parade, issued with a giant headdress made of peacock feathers, forgot all about Depression and went prancing off into the balmy sunset.

I presented myself to the guard at the gate of the hospital. English was his second language and it took a while to convince him that I needed to see one of the doctors inside. He seemed impervious to my depressed posture or my tears. Then, with nothing in his bearing that indicated a change of heart, he let me through the gates and pointed out the building where I should present myself for assessment.

After a short wait in the corridor, a psychiatrist emerged from a nearby room and asked me to come inside. She took a fairly comprehensive psychiatric history, recorded a few personal details and asked me a number of rather innocuous questions that I can only assume were part of a standard list for patients presenting with psychiatric symptoms. I remember being asked if I heard voices - presumably to rule out illnesses like Schizophrenia - and whether I knew what day of the week it was. Had I been anywhere else, I would have replied immediately that it was Sunday but I had so many misconceptions about psychiatric hospitals that I found myself thinking, "Don't, whatever you do, get this one wrong." I paused to double check my mental calendar that it was indeed Sunday before I answered that particular question.

The psychiatrist then moved on to ask some *DSM-IV* questions about depression. When she came to ask about suicidal thoughts and intentions, I became anxious and uncomfortable. I had experienced some suicidal thoughts but, at that stage, they were frightening rather than consoling. The word 'suicide' has such immense power to elicit emotions that we are aware that the mere utterance of its syllables is risky if there is more than one person in the room.

Avoiding taboo subjects serves to increase the power of the associated words. Obviously, there is a time and place for exploring taboos – very few grandmas want to dispense advice on finding your girlfriend's g-spot - and that is as it should be. But if someone in your circle of friends is depressed, the risk of suicide should motivate you to bring it up in conversation. Similarly, if your teenage daughter is losing weight quickly and behaving oddly about food, anorexia nervosa is something you need to talk to her about as a matter of precaution.

I responded to the psychiatrist's question about suicidal thoughts or intentions by saying, "I wish I wasn't around."

There seemed to be a safety in euphemism that diluted the gravity of admitting that the seed of self-annihilation had germinated in my mind. Although my experience with suicidal impulses changed dramatically over time, I experienced my first pervasive suicidal thought in a manner similar to an aggressive obsession. It was an intrusive, anxiety-provoking and irrational thought that I sensed would demand a response if it became persistent enough. It was certainly a significant factor in my decision to seek help at the hospital because it occurred to me that suicidality was a by-product of the intensification of the other symptoms and an indication that my depression was becoming dangerous.

After a few more questions, the psychiatrist put down her pen, raised her head and said, "I'm going to admit you." I think she was aware that I had numerous misgivings about psychiatric hospitals and she sought to allay my fears by adding, "The place you are going is called a neuroclinic and it is quite safe. Patients who pose a risk to other patients are in other sections of the hospital." She told me that I was likely to be in the clinic for between four and six weeks and suggested that I phone a friend who could take me home to fetch whatever I needed for the duration of my stay.

The first person I met, after the formalities of admission, was an extremely confident and affable fellow who was emerging from the internal quadrangle where patients were allowed to smoke. He introduced himself to me as if I had just arrived in a new and exciting city. He ended his introduction by saying, "Stick with me, and you'll be OK." But this did not have the reassuring effect it might have done had I heard it from a fellow countryman at a youth hostel in Munich who was attending the beer fest for the third time.

As it happened, I ended up in the same room as Harold, the neuroclinic concierge. There must have been something wrong with him but his backslapping bonhomie meant that I had no idea what that was. The clinic seemed deserted but while I was unpacking, some male patients gathered in my room to introduce themselves. They all presented as normal, if slightly dishevelled, people. An old man lay motionless on the bed opposite mine and I learnt from the others that he had tried to hang himself. Judging by his blank stare and morose lethargy, it seemed to me that he was still ambivalent about his unsuccessful attempt. After I had finished unpacking, I sat at the end of my bed and listened to the other patients talking amongst themselves, while Harold flouted the regulations and smoked Lucky Strike cigarettes.

He lit them with his Zippo lighter in a quick-draw manoeuvre that befitted a mysterious drifter who had ridden into town at sunset, tethered his horse at the saloon and then sat alone all evening drinking whiskey and patting his holsters ominously.

The Zippo lighter struck me as the symbol of his incongruity. Many psychiatric patients smoke, but the ones I have met are generally trying to alleviate something like anxiety or boredom, as if nicotine is over-the-counter medication. Some of them smoke with a visible sense of purpose: inhaling with chest-heaving intensity as the ash is dispersed irregularly by their anxious hands. But seldom does this sense of purpose have anything to do with being cool or hip. Zippo owners are either naturally cool or intend to render themselves such with their Zippo. My own attempts at coolness have involved the purchase and deployment of a number of Zippos with negligible results. Needless to say, when I was admitted to the neuroclinic I didn't think to myself, "Shit, I forgot my Zippo, now I'll never fit in." I had a sense that the concierge was hiding something but I had no idea what it took to be diagnosed with psychiatrically significant levels of coolness.

At dinner that evening, I saw all the other patients who had been in their rooms at the time of my arrival. None of them made me feel afraid. Some appeared sedated, some looked tired and others kept to themselves. The food was barely edible but this seemed by accident rather than design; and was probably because it was a government hospital with stretched resources. During the meal, a dark-haired girl in her twenties came rushing into the dining hall. She was wearing a lurid pink tracksuit and had tears streaming down her face. She crouched down in a corner, folded her arms and continued to cry. She seemed tormented. Her face had a desperate expression as if the source of her torment was some part of her she could not control and she didn't know how to rid herself of its influence. The corner provided only temporary sanctuary before she rushed out of the room, followed by a nurse who had failed to persuade her that she was being unco-operative.

On the way back to my room, I found her ferreting in the cigarette bin and I asked her if I could help. She looked at me with a pleading expression etched around her tearful eyes and said, "Do I have a future?"

Feeling utterly incapable of answering her question, I started by addressing what was obviously her immediate concern and offered her a cigarette. There was compacted ash under her fingernails from her attempts to scrape together enough tobacco from discarded butts to enable her to roll a cigarette of her own. I gestured to some overturned concrete building blocks on the other side of the quadrangle and suggested that we sit on them and smoke.

We sat in silence at first. There seemed no need for conversation as both of us were quite content to simply share the common ground of a habit, like two old fishermen on the same rock. When the time felt right, I decided to see if I could make a connection with her. Her body language had convinced me that I understood some of her pain. Her eyes reflected an emotion that I had seen in the mirror when my aggressive obsessions had overwhelmed me in London.

Sarah and I talked but not for very long. I kept losing her to whatever it was that was haunting her. I did manage to establish that she had, "a double called Isabel who keeps getting me into trouble". This other person inside her was not revealed to me during the course of our conversation and I made no attempt to bring 'her' out because my naïve fear and innate curiosity quickly reached an impasse in their negotiations. Oddly, I didn't feel intimidated by the idea of a double called Isabel for the entirely illogical reason that the only other Isabel I knew then was a gentle and loving person. But whatever her double was called, I had no idea what I was dealing with and there weren't enough cigarettes for the three of us anyway.

Much later that evening, I awoke to the disheartening sound of Harold singing along to his Discman. It was disheartening because he had a terrible voice. His lack of talent curbed neither his volume nor his enthusiasm, for which he showed no signs of remorse. Most dispiriting of all, he was unresponsive to the mood of his audience.

"Um, Harold, it's not really the time to be singing. I wonder if you could, ah, tone it down a little or, ideally, stop."

At this juncture, Sarah arrived looking for answers.

"Andrew, do you think I have a future?"

"Sarah, hi. Are you enjoying the concert?"

Sadly, my sarcasm was lost on Sarah and my remark was judged with almost autistic literalism as an unsatisfactory response to her inquiry. As such, she repeated it mercilessly.

"Sarah, do you mind if we talk about that tomorrow. Would you like some cigarettes?"

I felt that a rhetorical question was the prudent option in this complex and volatile situation. With a crucial personal issue still unresolved, Sarah left the room with her habit. Harold continued to sing.

Fly Fishing For Sharks

Harold the concierge yielded surprisingly quickly when I went over to his bed and, after complimenting him on his voice, asked him to stop singing. My sarcasm, although more subtle this time, was also lost on him. It turned out that all he was looking for was attention.

After a five-minute pause, Harold began exercising. This display of physical prowess included press-ups, other types of ups, martial arts lunges and kicks, as well as the odd taunt to an imaginary opponent which, thankfully, even he knew was not actually in the room spoiling for a fight. His physical activity was no more conducive to slumber than his vocal activity. I was wide awake by this stage so I decided to engage Harold in conversation with the intention of establishing why he was at the neuroclinic. I knew I would have to avoid direct questions and I knew I would have to start soon. In an ominous development, Bongani the Motionless was starting to stir on the other side of the room and it occurred to me that this time he planned to place the noose around Harold's neck, as opposed to his own.

Harold did not disappoint me as I started asking him about his life outside. He told me in hushed tones of his work for the government in elite military units and then later as a member of the intelligence agency. His testimony was sparse on dates, names and places because, of course, it was all classified information. Silly old me for asking for details. Harold was proud of his ability to defend himself from all manner of assailants. Apparently, he had been forced to kill someone who attacked him one night while he slept in his car on the side of the road. Harold, who more than most people knew the importance of an honourable burial, dug a grave on the same side of the road where he had slept. He then interred the unfortunate victim of his vigorous self defence and went back to sleep. Harold's training as a secret agent could have done with a few courses on incriminating evidence.

He ventured details of the scene of the crime. It was on a deserted coastal road about five kilometres from my parents' house in Cape Town, to which I would shortly be returning. Just before I began to get uncomfortable, I remembered that Harold was in the same hospital as me because he was ill. We were sick in different ways – Harold was suffering from delusions about his career and I was clinically glum – but something was wrong with both of us.

Harold's military and intelligence exploits were real to him but his life in the real world was complicated by his lack of insight into his delusions. If his illness was episodic like mine, he might experience periods of time when he realised that his life bore scant resemblance to James Bond's or Rambo's. The prosaic reality of this temporary lucidity must be distressing in its own cruel way.

I grew obliquely fond of Harold as we talked because it dawned on me that despite his repellent coolness and love of song, he was largely harmless and superior to a compulsive liar who is fully aware of his serial mendacity. At the end of the conversation, Harold suggested we exchange numbers in case he was ever in Cape Town. Not surprisingly, he fancied himself as a ladies' man and wanted to introduce me to Cape Town's nightlife. He was also a talent scout for a modelling agency, see, and this no doubt lent a certain durability to his harassment that it would otherwise have lacked. My telephone number ends with two ones and a two. The one I offered to Harold didn't. I'm sorry, but I was not going to spend an evening watching him empty a karaoke bar.

Chapter XVI

I'm looking for a book on cat massage

I was in the neuroclinic for only a couple of days. The panel of psychiatrists and staff who reviewed my case said that they agreed with the diagnosis made by the doctor who admitted me and that a four to six week stay was likely. However, they did suggest that if I had access to private healthcare, I should think about leaving Grahamstown and returning to Cape Town and seeking treatment there. I had admitted myself and was thus free to check myself out at any time. This was not the case with Harold who was admitted by a third party so required the panel's permission to continue his undercover work.

Once I had spoken to my parents and my psychiatrist, I took the decision to return to Cape Town. Phoning from a psychiatric hospital to which I had been admitted for depression gave me a sense of legitimacy about what I had known to be true but unable to describe.

Nothing in my mother's voice betrayed the sense of despair she must have felt when I told her where I was phoning from. Three months previously, it had seemed that I was stabilised enough to begin laying the foundations for a functional adulthood. Her hope now was that my psychiatrist in Cape Town would be able to put things right in time for me to return to Grahamstown to complete my studies; and avoid having to write off the entire year. In contrast, I had a horrible suspicion that a depressive episode that had manifested itself while I was already taking a high dose of anti-depressants, was not going to yield lightly to orthodox intervention; nor was it going to schedule its visit with the academic calendar in mind.

Much to the astonishment of many Capetonians, Table Mountain failed to cure my Depression. For those who have not been to or seen pictures of Cape Town, many of its suburbs are on the slopes of a mountainous peninsular, the most famous feature of which is Table Mountain. The mountains rise very dramatically from either the ocean or the flat stretch of territory that extends inland towards other mountain ranges of similar grandeur. Driving around the peninsular or approaching Cape Town from inland, provides views and photo opportunities that would enable an eight year old with a disposable camera to produce a marketable coffee-table book. It is perhaps not surprising that this scenery is invested with almost talismanic properties.

Many people fall into the trap of thinking that if they lived in the presence of natural beauty they would be able to cope much better with things in their lives that they consider unsatisfactory. This might be true for a small minority of people but repeated exposure to almost any pleasant stimulus will eventually result in a decreasing amount of pleasure. The rate at which this occurs will differ from person to person but very few Capetonians could honestly say something like, "If it wasn't for Table Mountain, I would never have survived the divorce." Living in a beautiful place is a wonderful ancillary benefit if the other important things in life are largely in place but it is not a substitute for those.

Due to the socio-economic effects of the *apartheid* period and, more recently, attempts by the post-*apartheid* government to encourage migration to Cape Town, one of the world's most beautiful cities has some of the world's most wretched slums. I would be interested to see the results of a representative survey of the residents of these slums that asked the following question, "To what extent is your crippling poverty alleviated by your view of Table Mountain?"

Fly Fishing For Sharks

The treatment for a Major Depressive episode that does not respond to SSRI anti-depressants is a hit and miss affair because the science of treatment-resistant depression is still young. A layman's description of the process would be to say that if the pills you are throwing at the problem are missing, then throw other types of pills until some of them start hitting. If the Depression is co-morbid with treatment-resistant OCD, just keep throwing. I was treated like royalty by our local pharmacist.

"Mr Alexander! Gosh how nice it is to see you. Do you need a repeat of your medications?"
"Yip, the whole lot please."

I would usually walk out of the pharmacy with a bag of merchandise comprising the sort of goods that muggers give back to you: anti-psychotics, SSRI anti-depressants, tricyclic anti-depressants, mood stabilisers, tranquilisers and anti-perspirants, if I was feeling impulsive. The highest number of different types of pills I was taking at the same time was only four but that was quickly dropped to three when I started writing poetry about the tranquiliser Valium. The psychiatrist said I couldn't have any more until my poetry improved but I suspect he thought I was developing a dependence on them.

"Have you ever tried to find something that rhymes with benzodiazepine?" I asked him indignantly.

'Alpine' is no good because the last syllable of Valium's chemical name is pronounced *peen,* and I have never liked the words 'latrine' or 'semi-evergreen'. Suffice it to say, you can only use the phrase, "Hey, chill out man" and expect results by insisting that whoever needs to calm down, must also take a Valium.

I never did go back to Rhodes University in that second half of 2002. By the time I felt well enough to return to university, I also felt that I would not be able to catch up on the work I had missed and go on to pass my final exams. The fact that I had Atypical Depression was somewhat of a blessing because I slept so much during the worst months. On some days I slept for up to eighteen hours and, while there was obviously an element of escapism in this, Depression must also have played a part because I made no use of sleeping pills or other tactics to induce such remarkable somnolence. Most depressives struggle to sleep and I can only imagine how difficult it is to have almost no respite from the distressing emotions and thoughts associated with the illness. Although I hadn't heard of 'learned helplessness' at the time, I was aware that my ability to mount coping responses to life's challenges was heavily comprised by Depression.

As I indicated earlier, learned helplessness was a dominant feature of my experience with Depression. I hypothesised that this was linked to how difficult it was for me to mount effective 'fight or flight' coping responses when my panic mechanism was activated by the obsessional thoughts associated with OCD.

The sense of helplessness was particularly acute with delayed-onset aggressive obsessions implicating me in other people's deaths. This was because I could not physically check the scene of the imagined catastrophe; hence the compulsive mental reconstructions could go on for weeks before I felt sure that nothing had happened. When I first came across the concept of learned helplessness, it seemed to provide an explanation for my first suicide attempt and I was struck by the notion that I had received some memorable lessons in helplessness from OCD. I am sure that helplessness can be unlearned but I wish it was as easy as my experiences of unlearning Chemistry.

Fly Fishing For Sharks

A particularly illustrative example of learned helplessness happened one evening during a depressive episode when I woke up at an odd hour and was finding it difficult to fall asleep again. I shuffled through to the kitchen in search of a snack, perused the contents of the fridge indecisively for a while and eventually decided to cut myself a few slices of gouda cheese. I took a knife from the cutlery draw and, brandishing the gouda in my left hand, I went to fetch the wooden cutting board from its usual resting place on top of the microwave oven. Seeing that it was not there, I looked around the kitchen and spotted it hiding under a small pile of unwashed plates.

For about thirty seconds I stood in the middle of the kitchen staring at the cutting board and the unwashed plates, as if the solution to my problem was not immediately obvious. The whole ridiculous incident ended with me returning the cheese to the fridge and the knife to the cutlery drawer and shuffling back to my bed feeling defeated and underfed. I was reading myself back to sleep about twenty minutes later when, with a mixture of confusion and disgust, I asked myself why I hadn't just taken the dirty plates off the cutting board. Removing dirty plates from on top of a cutting board is not at all difficult, as I discovered when I returned to the kitchen. But that is my point: the fact that I stumbled in the face of such an insignificant obstacle was an indication that my capacity to mount effective coping responses had been compromised.

The cheese example was faintly amusing but the underlying malfunction became considerably more serious in the face of genuine challenges. Learned helplessness took its toll on my ability to function in most areas of my life and was entrenched by either failure or a lack of the confidence, courage and motivation needed to face a particular challenge in the first place. My lack of engagement with the world also played a role in compounding the Depression of which it was a part; and, as the failures and early withdrawals mounted, I begun to despair about the future. This increased my vulnerability to relapses, during which suicidal impulses grew progressively more intense.

In early 2003, I began looking for work in Cape Town. The depression had lifted towards the end of 2002 but I was not interested in going back to Rhodes University for another year to finish my postgraduate course. I had a large student loan to repay and I was reluctant to make it any larger. Also, I was tired of coming down with something psychiatric and having to return home with a piece of paper signed by a doctor rather than a vice-chancellor.

At Rhodes, my intention of pursuing a career in investment banking had still been alive. When I was eighteen, this career path was simply a manifestation of relatively harmless naivety and healthy ambition; but eight years and some CV-changing illnesses later, I should have known better. Now, however, I admitted to myself that becoming a derivatives trader was the adult equivalent of my childhood ambition to follow in the footsteps of Batman. I found myself with no idea as to what I wanted to do. I also had no idea that in my position, deciding what I wanted to do did not necessarily mean that companies wanted to hire me to do it.

People tend to be tentatively sympathetic about Depression, viewing it as the medical equivalent of crying wolf. But if you are really looking for stigma, try long-term unemployment. I sent off applications, registered with some employment agencies and did a bookkeeping course but, in truth, I did not work very hard at looking for work. I was feeling sorry for myself. I was scared of a repeat of my job-related meltdown in London and a growing sense of fatalism about the future was corroding my motivation.

Fly Fishing For Sharks

People often exaggerate the importance of the work that they, their children or their partners do by the use of vague yet exciting terminology. When a parent says, "My son's in the catering game," I make a point of asking for details because if he is an award-winning chef, you can be sure mom or dad would have been more specific. The word 'game' is a useful cover if he happens to be a cutlery salesman because it conjures up images of strategy, suspense and victory. Are till operators at late night convenience stores caught up in the thrills and spills of the currency game? Are coalminers lured into the bowels of the earth because of the irresistible lure of the energy game?

Companies can be just as obfuscatory as people. I once applied for the position of a 'wired warrior' at an internet bank because it sounded interesting and a lot more fun than packing fish in Alaska. It turned out that the term 'wired warrior' was a catch-all phrase for the entire staff and that I was being considered for a position in the bank's call centre. Most of the questions in the interview dealt with my previous work experience so I was not surprised to be told that they found me "too ponderous and slow" for that particular division of their army. I was also asked if I could "think outside the box". That is a loaded question if there ever was one. I was hardly going to reply, "No I can't. I'm amazingly unoriginal, hide-bound by traditional thought patterns and wedded to a narrow worldview." The bank eventually went into liquidation. I imagine pesky 'inside-the-box problems' like sustained losses, mounting debt and lack of customers did not eventually succumb to lateral thinking.

In May 2003, my uncle, John Osterberg offered to pay the outstanding amount on my student loan which, at that stage, was all of it. My father had been covering the interest payments while I looked for work but the principal was untouched. John's selfless magnanimity not only lifted a burden from my shoulders and those of my parents, it also revealed how the startling generosity so familiar to those who know and love him was unsullied by ulterior motives and driven by his commitment to family and his capacity to love. With the disclaimer that the following assertion uses a necessary degree of semantic leeway, I have been lucky in love with my family and friends.

I secured my first job through someone I knew. I had always thought that the expression "it's not what you know, but who you know" was used by individuals implying that they knew from a young age how futile it was to study. It was chastening for me to realise that my inferences had been wrong and that these individuals had stumbled across a platitude that I had foolishly ignored. In this case, the person I knew was a beautiful and extremely competent publishing executive whose brother had studied with my sister at Oxford. Lynda knew that I was forlorn about being unemployed and was dimly aware that I liked books.

The chain of bookstores that eventually hired me only advertised vacancies for counter staff within the industry and Lynda was kind enough to inform me that a position was available. I had never fantasised about standing behind a counter and operating a till but eight months of unemployment had played havoc with my idea of a lucky break. I had to make it on my own through the CV lottery and past the interview; but Lynda's inside information transformed my job-searching endeavours from fly-fishing for sharks, to something more along the lines of persuading your infuriated mother that you lied your way into watching *Basic Instinct* because of a profound devotion to the works of Michael Douglas – that is to say, tricky, but certainly not impossible. My official title was "bookseller," but when I got the job, I did not tell people that I was now in the 'reading game'.

Fly Fishing For Sharks

The first few months at the bookstore were surprisingly bearable. The bookstore was in a gargantuan shopping centre that abutted a major highway and my commute was against the traffic. During lunch hour I would stroll around browsing in shops, or read newspapers and magazines in a little coffee shop that tolerated smokers. In those early days, the strange requests of customers were still a source of fascination to me and it became a challenge to trawl the store's computers to help a customer find the book they were looking for.

I learnt, to my astonishment for instance, that a book on massaging cats had been published. In fact, about twenty-five titles on the subject had made it to the shelves. In the process of my discovery, I watched my customer - a little old lady - regain some of the lost vitality of her youth. It crossed my mind that her cats might not be similarly reinvigorated by the news.

One day, a woman in her early thirties bounced up to the counter and announced, "I have been sent here by my friend because I don't get embarrassed by anything," with what I thought was a misplaced sense of pride. I wanted to say, "Oh fantastic. I look forward to becoming embroiled in a fruitless search for a book about some obscure and embarrassing medical condition whose name you've forgotten. Let me guess, the title escapes you, but the book is yellow and the author's first name starts with a P."

She said, "I want you to show me everything you've got on vaginisms," as if all reputable bookstores had a few shelves devoted exclusively to this subject.

At least she knew the name of the condition, if indeed it *was* a condition. It was extremely unlikely that we had anything on vaginisms at all but I was more concerned that her inquiry obviously dealt with the vagina and all our female counter staff had fled to other areas of the store.

"Ma'am, I'm not familiar with the word but let me just check our computers and run a few searches."

"Oh, it's actually more common than people think."

As each search yielded no results and I started running out of options, beads of sweat formed on my forehead as I considered the prospect of having to ask this customer for details of the condition in order to refine my search.

"Ma'am – ah - sadly our computers have not found any books on the topic. Are you sure you have the correct name? Or the correct spelling for that matter?"

"Yes, it's definitely vaginisms. V-A-G-I-N-I-S-M-S."

With a grim sense of foreboding I asked for details, at which point the customer shed her thick skin and begun to show distinct signs of embarrassment. My colleagues were now giggling behind the pillar at the centre of our circular counter.

I opted for the direct route, leaned over the counter and asked, "Does it have anything to do with the vagina?"

With the ice broken, she called me aside and explained that her friend had just got married and was having sexual difficulties because her vagina contracted each time her husband attempted to insert his penis into it. This malfunction was apparently resulting in less marital bliss than the couple had anticipated and the situation had recently been declared a crisis.

If I had been more worldly wise, I would have realised that it was my customer who was afflicted with an uncooperative vagina but this knowledge would hardly have made the situation any less awkward. After a few more keyword searches, I gave up and suggested that my customer's "friend" consult a doctor.

The next time I visited my doctor, I mentioned the incident to him and found out that the correct word was 'vaginismus'. In fairness, my customer was almost right and was to be commended for her proactive visit to our bookstore. I felt a little bit sad that I had had to send her away empty handed and had been tempted to tell her that there were plenty of books on how to massage pussies that might help her "friend's" husband out of his tight spot.

Chapter XVII

An ample-bosomed nurse with kind eyes

I was making small talk one day while writing this book, with a woman from the publishing industry. On hearing my description of its content, she said, "The misery memoir is very popular these days."

At first I thought that I was lucky to be writing in a genre that was popular. Then I realised that misery is one of the world's most competitive industries. And then it dawned on me that not only do I have scant reason to be miserable, but I am way behind in the equally tough business of defeating misery and turning it into inspirational recovery.

I had recently been going through an issue of *National Geographic* and had come across an article about a blind person who had climbed Mount Everest. A blind guy! This struck me as not only a challenge to those of us who can see, but also to other blind people because I saw no evidence of a guide dog in the accompanying photograph. Then it seemed that everywhere I looked people with no legs were playing tennis, victims of terrible abuse were thriving, the downtrodden were treading up; and hoards of courageous individuals were refusing to be victims.

I once heard a pastor give a sermon in which he voiced the opinion that the word 'victim' should be eradicated from the dictionary. He had met a very courageous blind boy whose triumph over adversity had been enough to convince him that no-one else should be a victim again, forever and ever, amen. This was normative thinking at its simplistic worst. It was also an ironic thing for a pastor to say. If the human race was not irredeemably a victim of Adam's original sin, then why did God have to love the world so much that he sent his son to die on a cross? Christianity doesn't work unless we all fall victim to our corrupt natures.

The pastor wasn't the only one shouting, "The last paraplegic up Everest is playing the victim." Secular conventional "wisdom" is coalescing around the view that you are playing the victim if you don't recover and thrive when life knocks you down.

I don't doubt that some people do play the victim but the label is applied too readily and with too little information. I have been accused of playing the victim by a good friend. When she said that, I felt ashamed that she thought of me in that way but I struggled to identify which of my behaviour patterns had led to the accusation. I didn't know how I got into the victim game, and I didn't know how to get out. Victims are often frightened, in need of someone to talk to and just trying to make sense of their predicaments. I met these criteria the night my friend made her comment because I was struggling to hold down a job. If I was playing the victim, I was also in need of help. What I didn't need was the isolation and guilt of another stigmatising label.

Whether or not I was playing the victim and becoming the author of my own misery, I started to become miserable at the bookstore. On the first day, my manager had given me a tour of the store which included a brief look into the room in which the store accounts were prepared. As soon as I saw the calculator, the computer and someone counting cash and credit card slips, I felt extremely fortunate that I had not been hired to perform this task on a daily basis.

I was thus apprehensive when, a few months later, my manager announced at a staff meeting that I was to learn the accounting function. She had no idea about my OCD because I had said nothing about it. The medication I was taking at the time allowed me to drive to work without thinking I had killed someone on the way, stack the shelves without thinking the books had blood on them and operate the till without quadruple checking each stage of the transaction.

I was slow on the till but in an eccentric way that resulted in the nickname "J-slow" rather than a petition for my dismissal. (Few things in life have surprised more than being assigned a nickname derived from the one used by the fans of Jennifer Lopez.)

I was coping with life as "J-slow" and eager to remain employed. Although nervous, I tried to remain positive about reuniting OCD and accounting after their amicable divorce at the end of my first year at university. I think that the problems at the bookstore stemmed from the fact that I was dealing with real money, rather than the pretend money of Widget Trading Co. (Pty) Ltd. The medication ensured that my new role did not lead to the rapid disintegration that had occurred in London.

After a couple of months preparing the store's accounts, however, I was once again showing no promise in cash management and being fired looked possible. The dynamics of my difficulties were no different to those I had experienced altering account balances in London or writing Maths exams at school. I was consumed with the obsession that I was continually making mistakes and, as a result, I spent too much time compulsively checking my work in a classic OCD cycle of dysfunctionality. The pressure of a time constraint meant that the tension between the need to check and the need to continue was additionally high which magnified the level of stress.

The end result was less traumatic than in London and it manifested itself over a much longer period of time. It was less traumatic because the relapse took the form of a slow onset of Depression, rather than a harrowing paroxysm of aggressive obsessions. However, the reality of delay rather than prevention indicated that the medication did not offer the psychiatric stability I had hoped it would. This made me even more timid about formal employment and the outside world. The infection from the Komodo bite continued to spread.

I took some steps to counteract the decline. I visited my psychiatrist and explained that I was worried about the situation. He prescribed some mood stabilisers to halt the depressive relapse and raised the dosage of the anti-psychotics to alleviate the OCD. I implied to my manager that I was under strain and she split the banking task between myself and another employee. But after reaching the end of my tether, I applied for a position at another store within the chain that had a permanent accounts clerk and accepted the offer of a transfer in the hope that I had found a solution to my predicament.

I have no idea why I did not improve at the new store. I knew that I was in dangerous territory when I started taking tranquilisers after dealing with particularly difficult customers or with phone queries from people with time on their hands and a list of obscure titles. There was an element of frustration in my response. There was a desire to avert drenching the next difficult customer in a shower of invective. And there was even a longing for the temporary fog of nonchalance that Valium provided. But the dominant impulse was to stop the daily insult of existence from hurting so much.

I made an appointment with my psychiatrist, who sensed my desperation and admitted me to hospital on the following day. It was August 2004, and I had been employed for about a year. During this time I had learned that I was still allergic to accounting; that the customer is a despotic and tyrannical king who is almost always wrong; and that matrimony is drained of some of its holiness if the bride has a history of vaginismus.

Being admitted to a psychiatric facility is much easier when your doctor has phoned in advance and a medical aid company has agreed to cover the cost of your treatment. This time there was no suspicious security guard. Instead, there was an ample-bosomed nurse with kind eyes and a background in psychopathology. She had permed hair and a smooth, monotonal voice that would have been patronising if she had spoken any slower. Her voice was accompanied with empathetic nods of the head, a commitment to eye contact and a permanent smile. She made me feel like a seven-year-old boy who is flying unaccompanied and speaking to his first airhostess.

"Good evening, Andrew, and how are you at the moment?"

"Fine thanks, Nurse Jeanie."

I spoke much like a seven-year-old as well.

"Did you enjoy your dinner tonight Andrew?"

"Yes, it was nice."

"That's good, Andrew. Now, if you need anything tonight, I will be just down the hall at the nurses' station."

"OK, Nurse Jeanie."

The hospital was a private clinic and thus, unlike in the government neuroclinic, the length of a patient's stay was determined by a more commercial assessment of treatment needs and available funds. I was in the clinic for three weeks but even if the money had been available, I don't think a longer stay would have made a great deal of difference. I entered the clinic with the hope that it was the custodian of the secrets to permanent recovery. The last time I was admitted to a hospital by a doctor, I had problematic wisdom teeth and, by the time I was discharged, my dental problems had disappeared along with my wisdom teeth. Experience had shown that psychiatry does not conform to such a simplistic paradigm of treatment but hope is about willing the future to be different from the past.

The clinic was a business with committed staff and good intentions but if any group of patients is going to thwart the objectives of a mission statement, it is a psychiatric one. I knew from Economics class that Adam Smith's "invisible hand" which was supposed to guide a capitalist economy, became very clumsy in the market for healthcare and the clinic was a good example of this. I entered a treatment programme that was too generic for the range of problems it was hoping to address.

If anything in the programme made me yearn for robust mental health, it was the weekly beading session. When I first sat down in the arts and crafts room, I looked nervously at the piles of beads and strips of fishing line and knew that my manhood was at stake. In times gone by, I had harnessed my illusions to seek the life of a bodybuilder and then a banker and although these were transient aspirations, they were driven by impulses that are foreign to the world of beading.

I raised futile objections to the lady contracted by the clinic to equip patients with elementary beading skills. I was already one of the few males on the programme and I feared that if I successfully manufactured either a necklace or a bracelet, I would be in danger of being declared an honorary woman. There is absolutely nothing wrong with being a woman. Unless you happen to be quite content as a man. I made a prominent display of placing my box of Marlboro Reds next to my beading mat - just in case there was any doubt that I was firmly in touch with my masculine side. Punctuating my efforts with the odd manly grunt, I produced a necklace and a bracelet of deliberately poor quality. I admit I was being ridiculous but I hadn't felt like a man who would make his father proud for a long time - and I wanted to at least act like one.

Weekdays in the clinic began, not surprisingly, with breakfast. The first item on the treatment agenda was usually group therapy, during which patients were encouraged to express their problems in words. The session was moderated by psychologists and occupational therapists. This was to prevent a situation in which an anorexic girl received unsolicited advice on how to put on weight from a very rotund woman in vacuum-packed jeans, who was raised in a culture in which overweight women were seen as highly desirable. Such a situation actually developed one morning while I was at the clinic. It was so unexpected that the therapists were unable to prevent it entirely.

"You mustn't try to be skinny, men like fat women. If you eat lots of peanut butt…"
"Yes, thank you, Peggy…um…let's try to avoid value judgements."
"But I can help her to eat more. For example…."
"Peggy, that's very kind of you, but can we leave it at that for now."
"Ok, but…"
"Right, group, who haven't we heard from today?"

From time to time, we were corralled into a large room and put through an hour of drama therapy in which we were encouraged to express our problems through movement, mime and dance. These were some of the longest hours of my life. I hope these sessions were not taped and analysed by therapists at a later stage. I hate to think what feedback they would have given to my psychiatrist.

Patient: Andrew Alexander.
Diagnosis: Obsessive-Compulsive Disorder with co-morbid Major Depression.
Activity: Drama therapy.
Andrew exhibits little dramatic talent but it is clear that the frequent grimacing we observed during his 'Dance of OCD' was a manifestation of his tendency to internalise his anger. The stark dichotomy between his movements and the rhythm of the accompanying music reveals that the patient is unwilling to accept the limitations placed on his life by his dual diagnosis. During one particularly revealing activity, Andrew failed to a reach a rope signifying 'the future' which had been placed at the far side of the room by the drama therapist. He was thwarted in this regard by an imaginary pair of malfunctioning crutches that he chose to reflect the inadequacies of both his medication and his willpower. This obvious fatalism and victim mentality signifies that Andrew has never processed the loss of his placenta in childbirth and seeks to return to the safety of the womb. The patient should be monitored as a suicide risk. Lastly, Andrew often selected the same attractive female patient when the group was asked by the therapist to choose a partner. We have no idea what this means but subsequent fraternisation should be discouraged in line with hospital protocol.

The programme involved many other types of structured sessions that either attempted to explain why we had problems to begin with, or how we could avoid them in the future. Some sessions bore no relevance to any of us in the programme. A woman spoke to us about what it is like to have an alcoholic husband and kept repeating the phrase

"Shit stinks, but it is warm," to illustrate how people can get stuck in horrible situations. I understood what she was getting at but I would have preferred a level of insight that arose from years of study, rather than the type of crass generalisation I would expect from an aging stripper with a philosophical streak.

One of the speakers encouraged us to "Let go, and let God," when we had reached the stage where all human interventions had been tried and found wanting. This well-intentioned sound bite provided me with no solace, not only because of its glib irrelevance but also because we were in a hospital and patients deserve more respect than to be told that God will step in when medicine has run out of ideas. It would have been more therapeutically consistent and considerably more honest if we had been told instead that, in addition to being warm and stinky, shit also exhibits a reliable tendency to just "happen".

Chapter XVIII

I do not want this

During the eighteen months that followed my discharge from the clinic, I came to the conclusion that what I really wanted to do with my life was end it.

It wasn't the clinic's fault that I made the transition from being alarmed by suicidal thoughts to being tempted by them. I had resigned from the bookstore and had no intention of returning to a job that combined the boredom of traffic jams with the trauma of either accountancy or customers with vaginal complaints and tense cats. As such, I needed to plan my next step and this resurrected my haunting fatalism.

My reasons for attempting suicide were not particularly compelling to anyone except me. I was simply tired of not coping and the prospect of life as a cycle of relapses was unacceptable. I hated depression and I hated OCD. I hated the impunity with which they bullied me and the taunting threats with which they mocked my plans. Because they lived within my mind and I felt increasingly helpless, it seemed that that the only way I could neutralise them was by killing myself.

I made two suicide attempts. Both of them resulted from abortive efforts to study at UCT for a third, and then fourth time. My mother was working for the university and the fees were thus considerably reduced. The first time I withdrew from UCT within weeks; and the second time, within a day. Both courses seemed like a good idea at the time and both would have resulted in jobs that were better than the bookstore.

Both suicide attempts resulted in hospitalisation and electro-convulsive therapy. In the first case, my psychiatrist gave up on me. After years under his care, he reacted to my overdose by saying, "I don't do hospital visits." In the second case, my family gave up on the psychiatrist. He had picked me up the year before when the previous fellow had refused to come to the hospital.

Learned helplessness and the ghosts associated with UCT turned academic assignments into sources of desperate anxiety and reasons for leaving. Frustration, anger and fear helped me swallow the pills and, a year later, slit my wrists.

The first attempt was in March 2005. I overdosed on my prescription medication. Unlike the second attempt, the overdose was an impulsive act. The teaching certificate I was studying for at UCT was going very badly and I was becoming increasingly desperate.

I was watching the Oscars ceremony on TV in an attempt to relax one evening, a few weeks into the course. My head was churning with the implications of how paralysed I felt about attempting my first major assignment. With the mental and emotional fragility of learned helplessness, I was vulnerable to the most irrational impulses. In the turmoil of uncertainty, I came to a dramatic conclusion.

I said to myself, "If you can't handle this assignment then you can't handle life anymore. I think it is time to stop putting things off and kill yourself."

I said good night to my family and went to my room where I began writing a suicide note to them. It was surprisingly easy to write. All the things that I couldn't explain to them face-to-face came flooding onto the pages of the notepad. I was agitated rather than emotional as I emptied almost a month's supply of the drugs I was taking at the time onto my duvet. Each one had to be removed from its protective blister pack, so there was ample time for me to appreciate how many there were.

I swallowed about five pills at a time and when I had finished, I tucked the suicide note into my sleeping shorts and lay down in the expectation that I would soon be unconscious.

The pills took much longer to knock me out than I had anticipated – little did I know that the ones I had taken were designed to be reasonably safe in overdose. This gave me too much time to reconsider my decision.

After about an hour, I walked through to my parents' bedroom and told them what I had done. My mother rushed me to hospital where I spent the night in intensive care, followed by three weeks in the psychiatric unit where I underwent a course of electro-convulsive therapy.

The second attempt was a year later, in March 2006. It was a windy night and I waited until I was sure that everyone in the house was asleep. I don't recall being afraid but I do remember that my hands were shaking. There was obviously some adrenalin in my system, released in anticipation of the pain that was to come. To counter this, I went downstairs to the drinks fridge and got myself a beer. I sat on the edge of my bed and sipped this at a leisurely pace, listening to the wind. Beside me on the bed were a screwdriver and a new set of Gillette Mach 3 Turbo razor blades. I figured that I only needed one of them, and a screwdriver seemed the most appropriate device for prising apart the apparatus. Despite the adrenalin, I wasn't particularly emotional that night. I suspect that this was because I had almost no doubt at that stage about what I was planning to do.

I had written a suicide note to my family.

Dear Family

I do not expect you to understand this. For years now I have been trying to explain things to people, and I have come to the conclusion that my experience of OCD and depression is not accessible to anyone but me. My first and abiding wish is that you realise that there is nothing to be sad about. I have suffered too much emotional hardship for my ability to process it. Depression and OCD are simply illnesses categorised by extreme emotions. I understand that you will be utterly devastated. I can only say that this decision gave that fact lengthy and agonised consideration. You have a right to be angry with me. All I can say is that I couldn't forever live my life as a favour to others, and in the end, I have the right to decide when enough is enough. What I can say is that there is nothing at all for you to feel guilty about. Nothing. Ever. You have all supported and loved me, and tried your best to help me through the tough times. Mom, you especially have suffered with me and done everything in your power to fix things. I ask that you try never to blame yourself for this. When I told you about how I felt last year, you said that if I took my own life, you would do so too. Please do not. What I would want is for you, once you have stopped grieving, to realise that I am happy now and free of pain. Celebrate what life I had because I do remember happy things. Wait for your grandchildren because they will love you as much as I did.

I came to UCT this fourth time with the intention of completing the course. I could not anticipate that the years of OCD and depression, and the setbacks they have caused, would deplete me to such an extent. I am too fragile now for the rigours of even an ordinary life. I am less scared by death than by the assignments I have to do, and the research project, and the challenge of an extra course. But if it wasn't this course then it would be something else, like a job in a bookstore or a move overseas or balancing the demands of having a family of my own. I can't just be a person who lives at home without a job, but that is all I feel capable of handling. That, you will agree, is no life at all, and it would become less of a life as time passed. I would feel too guilty, and even more so because I couldn't make my fragility accessible to you who saw me sitting around and sleeping my life away. I feel that I have fought a decent few rounds against this thing. I've grown weaker not stronger, and I fear that when I win a round or two, the illness changes form. OCD becomes depression, and depression becomes despair. I couldn't keep fighting. You might think, why did he not come and tell us how he was feeling about his course? Ask yourself this. What would've I done instead? What could we have tried that we haven't thought of? More medication would not have helped. I wouldn't manage on my own if I had tried to emigrate. I could've looked for work but given my history and affirmative action, that would have been a long shot. Yes I could have got menial work but it's too embarrassing, too boring, too depressing and too poorly paid for me to cover my medical bills, achieve independence and have any sort of quality of life. They say that lack of motivation is a key source of long term disability in severe mental illness. I was struggling with that.

Time to say something to each of you.

Rory:
I was so proud of you for finishing your degree. I can honestly say that I have never been angry with you. Sorry for any way in which I have hurt you over the years. Keep at it with your new job, you seem to be on to something good there. Please believe me that I was terribly unhappy and now I'm not.

Karin:

My dear sister. How proud I am of all you've become. You are an example to all of how to relate to difference in our society. Thank you for the advice and your love over the years. I also thank you for always putting such an effort into to my birthday presents while you were overseas all those years.

Dad:

Your stability and unjudgemental nature have given me so much peace during the illness years. Other types of dad would have caused me untold suffering but not you. I am truly sorry that you have lost your firstborn son, and I'm sorry I wasn't able to be the man I was supposed to be. Dad I couldn't keep wading through the muck. Never blame yourself; you, like me, were powerless and assigning blame is therefore fruitless.

Adam:

It has been good to know you. I so appreciated your mood raising power. The best of luck with your plans and ventures. You are the perfect husband for Karin, and I can see how much you love her. I hope you have a wonderful life together.

Mom:

I know you will see this as a failure on your part. I can only say from the bottom of my heart that it wasn't. You have tried everything and so have I. We laughed and we cried together. I love you deeply. So how can I do this, you scream? Because I know that it will get worse with time, this world weariness. Because I would cause you suffering for a long time to come as I lived on in this frightened, unhappy state. Because you know that as a free individual, the decision rested with me and that although you are my mom, I am Andrew with power over my own destiny, and the only one with true knowledge of my condition. I can't stop your

Fly Fishing For Sharks

pain, but I could stop mine. I am happy now. Just think of me as having a blissful sleep. Never blame yourself and never feel guilty. I would hate to think of you like that.

As soon as I had managed to extract one of the blades from the razor, I went to the bathroom. I took my shirt off and sat in the bath. I held the blade between the thumb and the index finger of my right hand. I made a few very shallow incisions in my left forearm in attempt to gauge how hard I needed to press to sever the veins in my wrist.

My first attempt to slash the left wrist was not successful but it was painful. I tightened my jaw, winced in anticipation and tried again, this time pressing considerably harder. A very clean wound opened up and for a brief moment there was no surge of blood. When the wound started to bleed, it was less dramatic than I had expected. I had cocked my hand outwards to assist the bleeding and, although much of the blood dripped straight out of the wound, some of it followed the inner contour of my hand and fell in large droplets off the end of my little finger. After many years of obsessions about blood and AIDS, the lack of revulsion I felt for my own blood was strangely refreshing. The dark intensity of its redness was almost beautiful against the faded white of the tub's old enamel.

Despite the wound, I had no difficulty slashing my right wrist. It was painful but it felt right. I cocked both wrists outwards, rested my forearms on my thighs and waited to die. In this position the flow quickened and the bottom of the bath started to fill with shallow pools of coagulated blood. Atheism provided a helpful - but not complete - source of solace as death approached. Unlike my previous suicide attempt, I was less troubled by last-minute doubts that my soul was damned. I felt powerful and in control for the first time in many years; and, perhaps more importantly, I had conviction that an unworkable future was being avoided.

195

At a certain point I broke out in a cold sweat, my hands started to shake again and I began to feel very light headed. I can only assume that this was due to the loss of blood. For as long as these symptoms persisted, it was very unpleasant and a huge contrast to my naïve expectation that I would slowly leave this world like an old man gradually falling asleep in front of the television. My memory of what happened next is patchy but I must have either lost consciousness or fallen asleep.

It was about six in the morning when I became aware of my surroundings again. My hands were resting on my stomach, but were now cocked inwards and the bleeding had stopped. The bottom of the bath was smeared with blood that remained wet, whereas the blood on my hands, stomach and legs had dried out, leaving the skin underneath feeling taut. As long as I didn't adjust my wrists, the razor wounds did not hurt.

I reacted to my unsuccessful suicide attempt with neither relief nor a sense of failure. I didn't feel lucky to have survived - nor that any special significance should be attached to the fact that I did. My emotionally clinical and coldly pragmatic assessment of my survival was that I did not slash my wrists in the correct manner and that I had not plunged the razor deep enough to sever the veins entirely.

You might ask why I didn't finish the job when I realised that my attempt had not been successful. I have asked myself the same question and I have struggled to come up with an answer. In all likelihood, I was emotionally exhausted and unprepared for the physical pain that I now knew was involved. Suicide takes motivation and courage despite the conventional wisdom.

Fly Fishing For Sharks

I have heard people say that suicide is for cowards. Convention is a suspect locus for wisdom, in the same way that commonly held beliefs often make very little sense. Despite my conviction that I had no future, I needed courage to slash my wrists and I needed more courage to remain seated in the bath while the blood seeped out of the wounds. After the manner in which the "knowledge" of a literal hell had warped my mind and catalysed my illness, I needed courage to look death in the face and know for sure it was not Satan welcoming me home. I needed the courage of my conviction that I had no future. I needed it especially in the moments when I paused before slicing my wrists open.

My trusty *Chambers* dictionary is of the opinion that courage is the quality that enables people to meet danger without giving way to fear. I think I am safe in assuming that the venerable *Chambers* lexicographers would not object to my using death as a temporary replacement for danger, for the sake of argument. Wanting to die is often understood by others as profoundly irrational or plain inexplicable and I can accept this. However, misplaced though it might have been, making the transition from wanting to die to taking my own life required that I did not give way to fear. In both my suicide attempts I was unsuccessful but the second time, I had more courage.

I started this book by telling you I was angry and bitter and I asked you to decide - after reading my story - whether I had a right to be. I had no idea that the catharsis of writing would purge even those emotions. It was an insecure question and I now realise that I don't need the permission of others to grieve my losses and process my pain. I have also learnt that anger and bitterness are important milestones on the road to acceptance and that, to accept something, you most certainly don't have to like it.

There is a song by the industrial metal band Nine Inch Nails entitled 'I Do Not Want This.' At the end of the song, Trent Reznor, the singer, repeats four lines of lyrics several times with progressively increasing passion and intensity. The last line always strikes me as a powerful statement about the human need for meaningful and significant lives. In his final repetition of the fourth line, he stops the music before leaving the last word ringing in your ears with a low-pitched scream. The effect is quite startling and more so because the line captures the essence of a universal desire. The line is, "I want to do something that *matters!*"

I have long wanted to do something that matters. I hope this book is it.

Fly Fishing For Sharks

Afterthoughts

I had every intention of finishing my story at the end of the last chapter because, from very early on in the project, I had planned to use those Nine Inch Nails lyrics to set the tone for the last line of the book. It seemed like a good idea.

I don't want to retract the sentiments expressed at the end of the last chapter but neither do I want to end that way. Of course, I *do* hope this book matters in some way but I was trying too hard to be profound - and that task is best left to stoned undergraduate Philosophy students.

On a more subtle level, my instinct to end with a number of loose ends untied stemmed from a desire to express the emotional discomfort that accompanies the fact that I am not convinced of my own recovery. I have certainly reclaimed lost ground from OCD and Depression since my suicide attempt in 2006; but that is what I thought before I left for London in 2000. The false confidence of what I assumed was mental health only made the lurid relapse that ensued more traumatic.

I started this book about a month after being discharged from hospital with the scars on my wrists still tender to the touch. I had been angry when I started writing this book: angry about the past I could not reclaim and angry, most of all, about a future which held only terror for me. When I decided that I did not want that future, I tried to kill myself. Although the psychiatrist attributed that act to the distorted perspectives of a mind warped by severe depression, I experienced a clarity of thought and purpose that night in the bath that was as sharp as the blade of the razor in my hand. The electro-convulsive therapy temporarily removed the suicidal impulse but left my views about the future intact. I had been struggling with this impulse for two years and I knew that it would be only a matter of time before it returned.

When the anger arrived, I did not resist it because I could see it eroding the helplessness that was the author of my despair and the root of my desire to die.

My anger helped me overcome the insecurities and doubt that had stymied earlier attempts to write my story. The sense of achievement and validation I experienced from doing something that I felt was worthwhile, made life so exhilarating that over the following few months I entered a state of agitated elation that had all the symptoms of mania except psychosis.

So exciting was my awakening after years in the wilderness that I didn't realise to what extent I was alienating some of my close friends and causing more anguish to my family with my aggression and uncharacteristic, risk-taking behaviour. I forged documents and lied my way into a bank loan to sustain my nightlife and sometimes went days without sleeping. Mania is associated with bi-polar disorder – formerly known as manic-depression – but my slightly attenuated experience of this psychiatric state was so invigorating that I made no attempt to moderate it.

It stills makes me chuckle that one of the symptoms of mania I found on the internet was described as "increased focus on goal-directed behaviour". Can you imagine the number of people who would like to be more focussed on achieving their goals? Of course, this aspect of mania has to be considered in the context of the other symptoms but I want to shake the hand of the first parent who leans over to his spouse in bed and says, "You know, honey, Jimmy's determination to set and achieve goals is really starting to

Fly Fishing For Sharks

worry me. If it is alright with you, I am going to encourage him to explore his lazy side."

Although I spent hours at the gym and began training for marathons again, I didn't write for two months and eventually my desperate mother arranged an emergency meeting with my psychiatrist. Her decision to do so was prompted more by the bank loan and the nights without sleep than any concern about progress on the manuscript. At the appointment, I made a fool of myself by insisting - at the top of my voice - that I was an alpha male who was being undermined by polycystic females. I had read somewhere that women with high testosterone levels were more at risk of developing ovarian cysts and had assumed, wrongly, that the testosterone also led them to try and thwart the aims of alpha males. My psychiatrist gave my mother a reassuring glance, as if to say, "I've seen worse," and promptly wrote out a prescription for lithium carbonate – the drug of choice for mania.

Three weeks later, I found myself lying in bed feeling frightened by life again, without my life-giving anger and with an unfinished manuscript that had been written by someone I now didn't have very much in common with. A less than consoling - and mildly ironic - fact that morning was that lithium was obviously a very effective psychiatric drug that had come into my life at a time when I could have used one that was only partially effective, like so many of the others I had taken. The other less than consoling fact was that I was acutely aware that I had a textbook case of 'decreased focus on goal-directed behaviour'.

The point is: having an unstable mind means that my life is characterised by an above-average level of instability. Combine that with the fact that life is anything but predictable and I would be unwise to declare myself well. In the absence of cures for mental illness, I have to be satisfied with learning to manage my instability so as to cause as little disruption as possible.

As far as I can tell, I had a severe case of OCD. An old taxonomy of the condition's varying levels of severity was used to rate patients on a scale from 1 to 14. When I was diagnosed, I was rated at level 12 or 13, depending on what kind of day I was having. In addition, I had a collection of symptoms that included most aspects of the OCD spectrum and one that I have yet to come across in my reading about the illness. I haven't heard of another patient who thought he might have stepped on a baby but I imagine he exists. I exhibited symptoms of scrupulosity or religious OCD, aggressive obsessions, contamination fears, ritualistic behaviour and the need to repeatedly check most of what I did in academic or work-related activities. Many patients fall into just one of these categories. The severity of my case with its wide range of my symptoms meant that I was a relatively unusual - and treatment-resistant - patient.

I mention all this because I want readers with OCD to know that the illness does not inevitably lead to a life of unemployment and depression. There is much that can be done about OCD and most of the people in my OCD support group are employed and coping with their symptoms. My case is instructive because its severity meant that any mistakes of management were generally disastrous and thus they serve as stark examples of how important management is to the prognosis and quality of life of someone with OCD.

Although my official diagnosis is treatment-resistant OCD, my biggest fear now is relapsing into Depression. I believe that my current state of affairs was not inevitable. If my doctors and I had managed my OCD better, I think that my subsequent experience of Depression and learned helplessness would have been milder. Major relapses are traumatic and terribly disrupting to life plans but many of my OCD relapses were theoretically avoidable.

Many OCD self-help books will tell you that you can beat OCD without medication. If your OCD is severely time-consuming and crippling, I don't believe that soldiering on without medication is at all advisable. My collapse at UCT in 1995, in London in 2000, and again at UCT in 2001 all took place on no medication. They were all major turning points in my life and contributing factors to the sense of powerlessness that informed learned helplessness and suicidality. In each case, the collapse happened over a matter of weeks but the recovery took months and the emotional damage was grave and long-term. And they were all primarily the result of errors of management.

Here is a list of what I have learned about the management of OCD. It is by no means exhaustive but I could have done with a list like this when I was diagnosed.

1. Use a psychiatrist, not a general practitioner, to manage your case.

2. Stay in regular contact with your psychiatrist. If your symptoms have not improved, tell your psychiatrist and ask him what he intends to do about it. If your symptoms get worse, don't let months go by while unhealthy neural pathways are entrenched in your brain – see the psychiatrist as soon as you can. Ideally, you want a psychiatrist who specialises in OCD or anxiety disorders.

3. Undergo a course of Cognitive Behaviour Therapy. This is not the panacea that some people think but it is useful and certainly helps you to understand and moderate your obsessions and compulsions. If you can't afford a full course, read *Brain Lock* by Jeffrey

Schwartz. It is the best guide to CBT I know of. Also, he has been on Oprah - not just any cognitive behaviour therapist gets flown to Chicago to sit on Miss Winfrey's couch.

4. Commit to long-term psychotherapy. It is not indicated in the treatment of OCD but mental illness is about so much more than brain chemistry. A psychoanalyst will help you to understand yourself and, at the very least, give you some insight into your behaviour and thoughts. Warning: insight does not translate into healing in the short-term. If you are going to be a regular with either a psychiatrist or a psychologist, be bold and negotiate a reduction in their hourly rate. This might sound unorthodox but persist because the savings add up.

5. If you are on a particular medication for more than 12 weeks and you see no improvement, get your psychiatrist to try something else.

6. If you do not improve on SSRIs – the typical OCD medications – ask your doctor to add an atypical anti-psychotic such as Risperdal or Seroquel to your drug therapy. Don't worry, taking anti-psychotics does not mean that you are psychotic; and you might have the wrong idea about that word anyway. Atypical anti-psychotics helped me to drive a car again and I recommend them in severe cases.

7. The side effects of the medication are meant to be complained about. You can always try another drug that might suit you better. Tell your psychiatrist if the medication is changing you in any way that you dislike. If you are a male and you can't get an erection, rend your garments and cover yourself in gravel. Afterwards,

go to your psychiatrist and complain. Viagra isn't just for active seniors.

8. Join a support group. No-one understands like a fellow sufferer; and empathetic friends are vital during tough times.

9. Don't pursue goals that are fiercely at odds with your condition. Although it is one of the hardest things to do, being realistic about how OCD limits your options in life is crucial to successful management. I wasted years trying to be a banker and it was a road to nowhere. It is a commonly held belief that where there is a will, there is a way. This isn't true: some things are not possible. Be easy on yourself about this aspect of management because it is terribly hard to accept that you have a condition that holds you back.

10. If you are religious, try to avoid people who tell you that your illness is as a result of demon oppression, satanic forces or some sin you have committed. OCD is an anxiety disorder and talk of the devil and demons is just going to give you a whole lot more anxiety and panic that you don't need. Although I no longer go to church, I have seen how the consolation of religion has helped people with mental illness. Ask God for guidance, perseverance, healthy neurons and a good psychiatrist but steer clear of people who claim to have a gift in 'deliverance ministry'.

11. Keep informed. Doctors often fail to keep up with the latest research and drug combinations. Use the Google Scholar function to keep up to date. Not all medical journals offer research articles for free but an increasing number of them do. Include the term 'free full text' with your keywords and this should help you to locate whole articles. An example of a typical search

inquiry would be 'treatment-resistant obsessive compulsive disorder pharmacological management free full text'. Google Scholar has an advanced search function which allows you to look for, say, only articles published after 2003; so make use of its refining capabilities. To find Google Scholar, just look above the keyword box on your country's Google home page.

12. Hope for a cure - but don't bank on one. Putting your life on hold until you are better is a risky strategy. Psychiatry is a long way from curing mental illness and it is more prudent to learn to manage your OCD than plan for the day when it all disappears. When I was eighteen I used to imagine all the things I was going to do, including investment banking, when OCD was out of my life; but before long, I woke up to find I was thirty and still dreaming. I want a cure just as much as you do but I want you to avoid the mistakes I made.

13. Watch out for Depression. As I have explained in this book, Depression is more subtle than OCD, so keep the list of symptoms I provided and watch your mood during tough times with OCD. Watch your mood especially when you have made progress with your OCD; and have time to sit back and realise what it has stolen from you. I believe that most OCD-related Depression comes from some form of learned helplessness. OCD is a good teacher of helplessness, which is why it is so vital that you become a good manager of your illness. This is hard in and of itself; but what is harder is when OCD is unmanageable because that is when the sense of helplessness is at its peak.

14. I am essentially out of advice, but I am reluctant to end at point number thirteen for the obvious, but entirely irrational, reason that it would be bad luck. At the risk of hubris, I would like to move from advice to wisdom.

Fly Fishing For Sharks

OCD is a misunderstood and cruel illness. Living with it is hard and often lonely. People will tell you to get over it. People will tell you that getting better is about will power alone. Friends might make light of your hardship and abandon you. You might be tempted to give up. You will have times when horrible thoughts will torture you or uncontrollable compulsions will make you moan with frustration. You will feel ashamed, humiliated and a failure - time and time again. However, while all this isolation and emotional pain is happening, while you confront setback after setback and loss after loss, something inside you will be growing. If you continue to fight the illness, it will grow bigger. In his book *The Road Less Travelled*, M. Scott Peck wrote, "One measure – and perhaps the best measure – of a person's greatness is the capacity for suffering." OCD is a form of suffering and I am sure that if you continue to endure it, one day that something that has grown inside of you will become great. This greatness may not be spectacular, it may not result in material rewards, but it will enrich you and those around you. It will also be evidence that you have truly lived. When you were diagnosed with OCD, greatness offered you a prize. Fight on and see what form that prize will take.

That about wraps it up from my side. You now know things about me that many of my good friends don't, not to mention my mother and father who will, no doubt, have preferred to remain ignorant of my erectile dysfunction; and that it was a mercenary copulator with whom I attempted to revive my flagging performance. I toyed with the idea of leaving the prostitute episode out of the book but I reasoned that once I had described myself as an atheist, some readers might have considered me beyond redemption, so I could hardly disappoint them with an account of good deeds. A commitment to honesty is inherently risky but the sanitised alternative was not an option.

OCD and Depression taught me to empathise. Sympathy means feeling sorry for someone; but empathy is a great deal more powerful. It might involve pity but it arises only when the observer makes an attempt to appreciate the reality of the sufferer. It arises from sharing another's pain and going to their dark places. Sympathy is a natural and spontaneous emotion for most of us. Empathy takes a conscious effort. Empathy comes with knowledge about others. Empathy is weakened by judgement and strengthened by the effort required to put aside what you think you know about life and other people.

Mental illnesses are often just the lurid extremes of emotions and cognitive processes that are common to us all. As such, the potential for empathy about illness in the mind resides in all of us. Superstition, ignorance and fear are at the root of society's often inadvertent isolation of the mentally ill.

I hope that the little knowledge that I have acquired through illness and written about in these pages will bring out the empathy in you if and when someone important to you starts to become different.

Fly Fishing For Sharks

A mother's PS

As you may remember, Andrew refers to me as Mum Quixote, not only because of my idealism, but also because of my regular early morning inspirations on how to tilt at any number of windmills. The entry in my school magazine perhaps captures the negatives and the positives of this trait – *committee of one gets things done*.

But after Andrew's overdose in 2005, this optimistic 'committee of one' had to admit defeat. I was powerless to stop the curveballs that life kept throwing at my son. But I run ahead of myself. Why set down any more of my son's story when he has done it so ably himself? Were there early signs that we missed? Do I have my own list of 14 points?

I think that I would have benefited from hearing a mother's story. I hope you do.

Andrew was born in Mowbray Maternity, Cape Town. My waters broke just after early morning tea on March 23rd 1976, and my darling mum, who was down from Harare for the birth, insisted that I have a boiled egg to give me stamina for the day ahead. Bruce had to negotiate the very bumpy detour via Hout Bay (as Victoria Road was being widened) but in the early afternoon we were delivered of a bouncing 9 lb 3 oz boy. Forceps had to be used, but his Apgar rating was high and aside from a short time under the lights for jaundice, he continued to thrive. The only problem he had as a toddler was a persistent post nasal drip and I was advised against food colorants (which is when I first started to make the lemon juice that many visitors to our home will remember as an Alexander trademark). He had to have grommets in his ear, as did in fact all three children - too much swimming probably didn't help.

Parenthood is truly a most remarkable experience. Not living near family, (my mum had died when Andrew was just six months old), I was fortunate in my co-mums. One such was Janet who read prodigiously on the subject and introduced me to Penelope Leach (versus Dr Spock), and to concepts such as babies reacting positively to human faces (hence all the faces stuck on to the inside of Andrew's pram top). Her son Benjamin was Andrew's great companion. Benjamin would ride his yellow plastic 'BP' bike at frightening speeds down the walkway to the newly built UCT men's residence, Leo Marquard, but Andrew was always more cautious. He was very strong physically though and loved to clamber on the rocks at Logiesbaai with his Dad and was very much part of the Alexander-Carter BMX outings on the rocks of Domboshawa several years later for example.

From a neighbour I discovered the British *123* activity series that he (and Karin and Rory subsequently) loved, and also Glenn Doman's *How to Teach your Baby to Read,* although I was somewhat chagrined by a UCT summer school series that cautioned that teaching your child to read was more about the mother than the child! Our playgroup was just the best, with six of us up and down the road from each other taking it in turns to host a morning three times a week. One of the mums dubbed Andrew the 'gentle giant' because he had a strong physique but was not aggressive by nature.

The move to Zimbabwe aged 5 was not easy for Andrew. 'Grown ups introduce themselves Mum,' said this little boy, tugging at my tennis dress as we adults sent them off to play at the bottom of yet another new garden. (From then on I have always made a point of introducing children, and still do.) Andrew left an idyllic Hout Bay pre-primary for a larger, more pressured equivalent in Harare. His portrait of the teacher there was of a person with a mouth almost as large as her head, but it was there that he made friends with

Fly Fishing For Sharks

Nick, and through him, Sam, and by the end of Grade I at Alexandra Park School, Andrew was again in a neighbourhood where he could ride to school and had a set of friends close by.

Were there any signs of anxiety at this time? When Rory read through this script, he made the point that he was the most anxious of our children and in fact Rory was. There were three instances in Andrew's early childhood that I can recall, but all of them seemed quite normal reactions at the time. Firstly in Grade II, because of his size and athleticism, he was picked for the school team. 'They (the supporters) scream so loudly during the race Mum,' he said, and was only persuaded to run in the age group above him by the headmaster who had a gammy leg and would have loved to have been able to run fast. Going by train to visit granny and grandpa for the weekend in Bulawayo was great fun and something we did a couple of times, but Andrew would always worry until his dad was safely inside the carriage, whereas Karin thought it fun that Bruce only just made it on to the train in time, having popped off to buy a magazine from the kiosk on the platform.

A third example was at the age of 12 or 13 when we were coming back from a holiday in South Africa. Andrew had read in some magazine on the plane that airfares in the year 2010 would be some astronomical figure. Not being able to afford to take his family on holiday worried him, (and that was long before Zimbabwe's hyperinflation!), and he came back to the issue often over the next few weeks. I mentioned this preoccupation to a fellow Monday-group mum and GP, Cathy, and she made the point that puberty is a point of high consciousness in a child.

There was of course the incident that Andrew writes about. I have gone over it again and again. I wish that it had never happened, that we had responded differently, but

211

psychologists say that if it hadn't been that incident, it would have been some other trigger because that is the nature of OCD. At the time, my friend Di remarked that sexual curiosity was absolutely normal and any abnormality that there was rested with the adult concerned. Another mum, with psychology training, recommended I phone all the families concerned and quash it before it was blown out of proportion, and that is what I did. I now wish that I had hugged him more, reassured him.

To get back to Andrew and his progress through life, his Grade II teacher thought he had a spelling problem, but his Grade III teacher thought not, and in fact he came 1st in his first formal school exams. We did however take him to a vocational psychologist who assessed the spelling problem as Andrew having the vocabulary of a far older child, and so she gave us a list of more mature books for him to read – *Stig of the Dump* was one that I remember and one that became a family favourite. Andrew was always at the top end of his class and won the Academic Cup in Grade VII.

My parents took us on great holidays. Not only was there the fun of it, but they were great believers in the broadening experience of travel, and in fact had taken all three of us to England and Sweden for six months when Daddy had his long leave in 1953. We took our three out of school for just six weeks in 1989, to take advantage of the cheaper skiing packages in March, and of Karin being eligible for a half price flight to America. The six weeks' absence in Form I did set Andrew back a bit, but the end of Form II saw Andrew again at the top of what was seen as a very bright set. His 'O' level results were a big disappointment though, both to the school and to him, and perhaps this was an early warning sign.

On the other hand, it often happens, or it had done to me, that one is good at Maths but as it moves into calculus and beyond, a different kind of aptitude is required. Andrew was part of the school group that went to the Math's week at Rhodes, and I had great confidence in his Maths teacher, so I suppose that is why Andrew's distress over Maths didn't signal something deeper to me. It was instead 'my' subject, English, that caught my attention in the first months of 'A' level. I had not really helped my children in any meaningful way at senior school, other than with a bit of French, and so it felt quite strange to sit with Andrew and his Shakespeare text one afternoon. I thought it would just be a case of showing him how to read in larger chunks to get the gist of the piece, but he found it impossible and wanted to understand each word before moving on. It was *Bleak House* though that finally led me to do something.

Andy Nimmo was that rare breed, a most empathetic and humorous teacher, and so it was to him that I went about Andrew's despair in the face of 900-odd pages of Dickens. 'I've taught it three times and never once read it cover to cover – just get hold of a good crib!' said he. When pressed, and when he saw the seriousness with which I posed my questions, he did pass the opinion that it was a particularly poor choice of set book for young men at 'A' level. I learned from a friend of a wonderfully gifted English teacher who took some private pupils, and it was Dawn who recognised that Andrew was a candidate for the more difficult Creative Writing paper and thus could opt out of the *Bleak House* paper. Andrew thrived under her guidance and so what might have been a warning light, obsessive checking, passed me by.

On the sporting field, Andrew still swum beautiful butterfly and ran a fast 100 metres, but it was rugby that was to become a passion in Lower VI. He became uncharacteristically aggressive, partly because he hated the fact that his school was a new school and did not have a great first XV. The courtyard between his bedroom and ours 'clanged' to the sound of metal on metal and grunts of male exertion as a group of seventeen year olds strove to build muscle. Friends' enthusiasm waxed and waned, but Andrew persisted.

I was most surprised when his Physics teacher, and a man for whom I had great respect, asked if everything was OK. He remarked that one of his friends had gone overboard on weights, and that it had been a sign of something deeper going on. We didn't see 'weights' as something to worry over, and Andrew's passion for rugby gave him much pleasure – from support for the All Blacks to the chance to tour with the school team to Messina. You will have read his prescient yet amusing account of that, a trait that was starting to define this young adult amongst his friends and within our wider family.

Having been fortunate to have been able to be a mum at home, with just part time lecturing stints, I re-joined the world of work in 1989 on a 60% week, before going on my own as a PR consultant in 1990. I really liked working from home because I was able to work and play as it were. I did notice Andrew's real concern about driving. I did get apoplectic (I'm not proud of throwing that cup of coffee!) over his not lending a friend (and at the time also Karin's boyfriend) the video of their 'A' level set work, *Antony and Cleopatra*, but I had NO idea of the life that was going on in his head.

I remember being really surprised by his question on the morning of his departure for UCT in February 1995, 'It's going to be alright isn't it Mum?' He had longed to go to UCT, longed to go back to Cape Town, and I wondered if the stress of the last minute run-around to get his student visa had unsettled him.

Fly Fishing For Sharks

As you know, it wasn't alright. Just 10 days later the phone rang, and this shaky voice said, not 'Happy birthday Mum', but 'Mum, there's something wrong.' He didn't really say what was wrong, but my friend Jane came on the line to say that Butch thought it was more serious than first year nerves. As fate would have it we were going down to my nephew's wedding in Jo'burg that weekend, and so we organised for Andrew to join us.

My birthday evening passed in a blur. It was the first time I had ever entertained clients - we had a table at the Des & Dawn Lindberg show at the Sheraton – and I was just so grateful for the show as it meant that I didn't have to make sensible conversation. All I could think of was how unlike my son this son had sounded.

As our car drew up at the Carters in Jo'burg, I hardly recognised the Andrew who stumbled down the lawn into my arms. As I held him, Di mouthed the words 'I think it is serious.' Bruce's instinct was that we needed some privacy and so he booked us in to a nearby hotel for that night, and we heard for the first time about the thoughts that were terrifyingly real for Andrew.

I bless Di (and Jane) for forewarning me though. How else would we have been able to absorb the litany of what was tormenting him, even as he kept saying that in his rational mind he knew it couldn't be true. It was so hard to not only hear him talk about the panic of driving to A-level exams but also to see the anguish as he recounted having to go back and check that he had not run someone over. UCT's showers and toilets were no worse I am sure than those of other student residences, but for Andrew they presented a minefield of contamination. And then there was his whole fear of having inadvertently sat on or stood on a baby.

We made an appointment with the Carter's GP first thing on the Friday morning, and I know that we were fortunate that she was a recent graduate, because shortly into the conversation she stopped Andrew and said that she felt we needed to see a specialist and it being Friday, she wanted to be sure of an appointment that day. We were booked to see a Dr Wessels at 12. He suggested we get a cup of coffee while he saw Andrew on his own first. Bruce and I went off to a coffee shop in the Sandton Medical Centre and sat close to each other on the seat. I could hardly swallow.

'Your son has a rare condition, Obsessive-Compulsive Disorder,' he said. That was the first of several times in the last twelve years that the air has seemed to go out of my lungs. 'Not MY precious son,' I screamed in my head. The EEG had shown tremendous stress on the brain. In his opinion, Andrew was not far from the desperation of taking his life. Tests also showed a high IQ but the information that 'this seems to happen to bright, sensitive young people' did not ease the shock.

There was a ray of hope, and that was medication by the name of Prozac. Prozac is so common now, but in 1995, I had never heard of it. He suggested that we arrange to stay in town until the medication had had a chance to work, and he also said that in a few weeks Andrew would see a big difference. He also suggested we look for a book called *The Boy Who Couldn't Stop Washing: The Experience and Treatment of Obsessive-Compulsive Disorder* by Judith L. Rapoport.

Thank goodness for Rescue drops! On the way to the church I tried to explain Andrew's condition to my brother. It was a conversation that we were to have with Karin & Rory, with others too, and it never got easier. 'The doctor says that it is like diabetes in the sense that it is a chemical imbalance and something you will have to live with for the rest of your life.' Of course, the symptoms are NOTHING like diabetes, but needing medication is the common factor and something I was going to forget, much to the detriment of Andrew in his early twenties.

UCT gave Andrew a leave of absence for six weeks, and we left him in the bosom of the Carters to drive home and sort out our lives so that we could be back in South Africa a couple of weeks later. Over the next decade, my life was to go on hold several times and I marvel at how family and friends (& clients) have just stood by us. In that March for example, Bruce and I were not at home to drive Karin to her United World College interview; and it was Karin who was there to support her baby brother at Sports Day and watch him go up as captain to collect the cup for Kudu, the house that both she and Andrew had been part of.

March 1995

Watching Andrew pack up his student life was one of the hardest things we ever did. He was so sad, so broken. I've mentioned Andrew's academic and sporting track record but if I was to isolate the essence of Andrew it would be in terms of his friendships, his ability to make people laugh, and to introduce them to the new ideas he's been reading about. He is much loved, and the six or seven guys who came out to the car looked as bereft as we all felt. The Dad of one of them later told me how much of an impact Andrew's ability to verbalise his vulnerability had meant. This vulnerability was something that came to mean even more to his peers in the years of the diaspora of Zimbabweans post 2002.

Bruce had to get back to work but Andrew and I stayed on a few more days to celebrate his 19th birthday with his friends; we went to see *Pulp Fiction* and then had fish & chips in the then relatively novel Waterfront. Andrew's eyes were full of tears as we flew out of Cape Town, the place that held such horrible memories but too the place that held good memories and that should have been the start of his adult life.

Back in Harare we saw a psychiatrist but he was a great disappointment. He did write out prescriptions, and that was of value as our family doctor heard only enough of Andrew's condition to dismiss the diagnosis as newfangled nonsense. In fairness to her, that was the reaction of most people I think. It was all very unreal to me too. I could only read those parts of *The boy who couldn't stop washing* that applied to Andrew's symptoms. Most of it was too much for me to bear at that time.

My friend Mim talks about people building a carapace, and I know that I did just that, because people can be very hurtful, often unintentionally. At a Bridge morning I organised to raise funds for the Karin's College trip to Israel and Palestine one lady called out to me, 'Would you mind talking to a friend of mine, her son has also gone mad.' Some people expressed concern that I was in denial about Andrew's condition, that it was about my vision of his future. 'What about **his** vision for the future?' I countered. Another thought he would have been fine if he had gone to boarding school. I had to try to discern what rang true, and to sail the uncharted waters as best I could.

When something like OCD hits if is often hard to see the golden threads in the tapestry of your lives but golden threads there were and still are, and lots of humour and fun too. One example was Andrew and Karin being at home together that April-May and learning to type. The machines they worked on at Speciss College were out of the Ark, and for someone as fastidious as Andrew was, the dirty keys were just too much. Much to the bemusement of his fellow learners, he solemnly donned surgical gloves and worked his way through the Pitman's manual.

Fly Fishing For Sharks

Another example was deciding to treat ourselves to the Grahamstown festival in July of that year, picking Sam up on the way. We loved it. But Andrew and I were also able to make contact with the remarkable warden of Founders Hall, Prof Surtees, and to take the decision that Andrew go to Rhodes the following year. Rhodes and College House were to become some of the best aspects of Andrew's life over the next four years, with friendships lasting on into 2007 that have been pivotal to his recovery.

An interesting aside is that we went on to Cape Town to check progress on a flatlet we were building at our house. At the roof-wetting I recognised Percy and Roy as the same artisans who had worked on the house in 1977. Under apartheid, they were both classified as 'coloured'and it was wonderful to hear the joy in Roy's voice as he spoke of his children's progress at Kronendal High School, a school that had been previously reserved for whites.

Karin, her friend Abi, and I got back from a glorious walk in the winter fynbos, and a swim with dolphins at Sandy Bay, to find a very moved Andrew. Form I placement was quite an issue in Zimbabwe. All three children had attended the government school down the road and so had no prior claim to the various private senior schools. Rory had just called to say that he had got into both St Georges and St Johns and wanted to pass his final choice past his big brother. With a generosity that was to become the mark of my eldest son, he advocated his rival school, St Georges, and that turned out to be the best of choices for his brother.

We travelled back via Kimberley and the 'big-hole' that had been part of my Swedish grandpa's prospecting life and we had our usual stop-over with the Carters in Johannesburg and used the time to check in with Andrew's doctor. It was great for me to be able to report that Andrew had persevered in sharing the driving, stressful as it was, even with Karin and I there as 'witnesses' to the fact that an accident hadn't happened. It was then back to Zimbabwe and to all the excitement and emotion of Karin's leaving for what had long been a dream of hers, Atlantic College in Wales. Six months later, it was Andrew's turn to go, to College House and Rhodes University.

The next four years were OK, and so perhaps we were lulled into false security?

Aside from the change from Accounts and a bit of a blip in June of his first year, Andrew's academic side was fine and in fact he was one away from top marks in both the final Economics and Philosophy exams. Most people did not know he had OCD. His girlfriend Gayle did, and was most supportive. He did not ask for any extra time in exams, and managed the 1700 km drive down to and back from Rhodes several times. He was Senior Student of College, and it was obvious from the friends who visited us in Harare that 'Stats' was one of the popular characters in res.

January 2000 saw Andrew down to 20mg Prozac a day and, under our new GP, was going to come off it entirely over a six month period. He did a teaching stint at a co-ed school and the headmaster told Andrew that he felt he was one of those rare beings, a born teacher. Andrew's comment was typically laconic. 'You have to discount the fact that there was an element of self interest in this praise - young male teachers are thin on the ground!'

In April, when we were at the coast after Andrew's graduation, the first reports of lethal farm invasions were coming through. A graphic image on Sky News was of a family's dogs grotesquely beaten on their front lawn. Farmers would gather in knots on the beach exchanging news, and some people were cutting their holidays short. For the first time, my heart was heavy as we turned North to go home.

Andrew decided to head for London. His visa came through in record time, and he left in the first week of June. Cooking a rare treat of Beira prawns on the eve of his departure, we had one of the then infrequent power cuts and had to use the gas braai. Perhaps we should have seen that as an omen, but Andrew seemed to love London. His great friend Heath, who not only knows all about the OCD history but is also very street-wise, had Andrew to stay, and advised him on the modus operandi of the employment agencies and so on. I revelled in his delight at emailing from an internet café, (a rare commodity in Harare at that time), at the British papers, at the great characters he had drinks with that day he worked as a postman, at his deep content at working in the lee of St Paul's.

But then came the phone call. Tube rides were nightmarish as the obsession of having knocked over a child, this time on to the rails, re-surfaced. I offered to fly over but he was adamant that he needed to come home. On August 1st he arrived, grey in the face and very shaken. He wanted to be hospitalised, to be cushioned from the world. Our GP decided the medication should be re-looked and advocated an old-school psychiatrist who would not medicate to the point of sedation.

The first consultation with the Serb was like being on the stark set of a low budget movie. He was unshaven and tensile, and his conversation was very much that of an anarchist. I was at that stage some way into my Feminist studies, and so was not as shocked by his Freudian outpourings as I think he hoped I might be. Karin however was outraged, and in hindsight I realise we should have pressed the 'Abort' button. His engagement with Andrew's mind, with the philosophy of ideas, did seem to stimulate Andrew.

Into the scenario came the warmth and fun of an unlikely friendship. We were asked to be a contact for a Swedish girl who had been to a small rural village in Zimbabwe on a student exchange programme and who had herself hosted a girl from that village in Stockholm. Emily was doing research for her law degree, and we saw quite a bit of her and in fact took her up to Troutbeck with us for a weekend. The three of us stayed on for a few extra days while I did some reading for my course, and I realised there was something more to their friendship when my son, a normally reluctant participant in a four ball, spent hours teaching her to play golf.

February 2001 saw a somewhat restored self-confidence in Andrew, enhanced by the fact that he had been accepted into the Economics Honours course at UCT. As fate would have it, Karin had persuaded Harvard to let her do a semester abroad and the two of them were going to share a flat in Rondebosch. I went down with them to settle in and Andrew was upset when I left, but I still didn't think to insist that Andrew needed the safety net of a script for Prozac.

The fall when it came a couple of weeks later was harder even than London. It was a friend from St John's days who found him slumped against a wall in Grotto Rd. We could hear that Karin was very shaken. For the first time, I think, she realised that her brother could get desperate enough to take his own life. When Andrew arrived home his body language was utter defeat. The Serb's talk of 'fighting it together even if it takes a lifetime' did not console him. He felt desperate, and I felt numb to the bone. My son's eyes took on a defeated and lifeless hue.

Fly Fishing For Sharks

We had planned to holiday in Cape Town that April but Andrew understandably didn't want to come. Bruce asked me to try and persuade him as he felt that it is only on holiday that there is any real time together. And so he came, but he slept much of the day and there was none of his spark, not even for Pete, a friend of Karin's from Atlantic College who was in Cape Town for a 21st, and whose gung-ho-ness Andrew had found endearing when he stayed with us the year before.

I realised I had to do something and asked Jane if she could recommend someone we could go to for a second opinion. We made an appointment and the three of us, Bruce, Andrew and I, knocked on a door in Campground Rd. But this time it was different. This time we did not expect much; we no longer believed there was any kind of real help to be found.

We were wrong. Kier was a calm presence and listened to the long saga, interrupting every now and then to ask a question. When it came to the recent history though, he could not contain himself. 'You could sue for malpractice! There has not been ONE example in the last 20 years of the Freudian approach working with OCD and someone with a severe case of OCD should never come off medication.' We were stunned, but was he right? The difference from the Serb was that he had facts to back up what he said, and we had to agree that on Prozac, Andrew had not only coped but got his degree, even if that Prozac existence had been a 'grey' existence.

We left with a prescription and the name of a cognitive behaviour therapist (CBT) and with a sense that our world had come back in to some kind of equilibrium. CBT could not start until the medication had kicked in, and we were advised to get hold of a copy of *Brain Lock* by Jeffrey Schwartz and to plan to be in Cape Town for at least six weeks. Once again, Elsa opened her home on the rocks of Llandudno to us, and once again Bruce set off home alone, this time with Rory. Karin lent me her lap top and I had the rare treat of large swathes of time with my UNISA prescribed texts.

CBT is best done with a co-therapist, and so it was that Andrew and I were in sessions together again. For the first time I had the model of the cortex and the basal ganglia explained. Andrew devoured the literature and had questions to ask. Feeling that life was now more manageable, in mid June we headed North once more.

We arrived just in time to travel to a farm 'in the path' of the total eclipse, and I am so glad we did. There all the expectation of the approaching shadow, the light that becomes eerie, but it was the silence, the absence of insect chatter and bird calls that emphasized for me the life-giving nature of the sun. I found myself shivering, and not just from the absence of warmth, and was put in mind of that Friday long ago when at that fateful ninth hour the world had darkened.

Our world was also darkening. The Zimbabwe dollar continued to plunge. The Reserve Bank stopped the facility of sending out student allowances. There was talk of drug shortages. Zimbabwe was becoming an anxious place to live, even for someone without an anxiety disorder.

A friend of ours came up on business in November and offered Bruce a job in Cape Town. Two months later, with heavy hearts we waved Karin back off to Boston, rented our house, put special costumes & paintings, books & puzzles in the storeroom and hugged our family a tight goodbye.

Fly Fishing For Sharks

2002

We crossed over the border in two cars loaded to the hilt, and almost didn't get much further! Bruce and Rory were in an accident and the scavenging panel beaters advised that we would be going nowhere for a week. Bruce was due to start work in a couple of days and so, armed with a letter from the traffic policeman, we continued our journey. As Andrew remarked, we must have looked like a family who had been thrown off their farm and had damaged their car on a gate post in the rush to avoid the mob of war veterans – certainly lots of fellow motorists must have thought that because we got many hoots of support.

Andrew went back to Rhodes to start his Economics Honours, Rory started his PPE at UCT and I worked on my dissertation, *A story that would (O)therwise not have been told* about a remarkable Zimbabwean who I had met though the Africa Book Development Trust. Bruce and I then had a truly marvellous time with Karin at Commencement – exploring Boston, being hosted in Cape Cod by old friends the Baldwins, meeting up with the Carters in West Virginia and visiting Washington & New York. I came back to an interesting position at the Faculty of Law and we were moving 'home' to Robinson Ave. Life seemed to be on a new trajectory.

Andrew's call was just such a blow. This time he was on medication. This time he had the support of the running club network, but this time the curveball that was thrown at my son came in form of *The Noonday Demon*[1]. Everyone tells you that Depression is treatable, although Andrew seems to have a drug–resistant form, but it is Depression that nearly broke my son and almost defeated this Mum Quixote.

---

[1] Book of this name by Andrew Solomon

This was the night of my first SOS to the handful of people I knew I could rely on to pray. Andrew was due to give the speech at Sam's wedding in three weeks, and he had been so looking forward to being there, to seeing 'the Carts.' The speech was written, but getting there seemed to present too Herculean a task. I would come home from work as early as I could. Andrew was usually still asleep but if he was up, he was so passive and his face was the colour of alabaster. We'd talk about how he so badly wanted to be there, but not if it had to be with him in the state that he was.

Kier was very concerned. He hadn't seen 'it' coming, and Andrew was on anti-depressants as it was. There was a real chance that another severe episode could turn Andrew into someone who was afraid to leave the house, yet if the median of his feelings was no worse, or even slightly improved, the trip might just be the shot in the arm Andrew needed. We were now eight days to take off and the dosages were doubled. Valium was a daily fixture. I hadn't told Di about Andrew yet. I just could not face the enormity of everyone's sadness, and of Andrew's in particular.

Two days to go and I got home to find Andrew looking at the picture of Sam and him white water rafting on the Zambezi. 'I think I should go,' he said. His ticket had been booked months before and he was travelling from Port Elizabeth via Johannesburg, and we were to meet up in Heathrow's Terminal 3. I landed first. The Johannesburg flight was announced and the luggage started to come through, but no sign of the suitcase for Karin that Andrew was carrying … My heart sank.

One of the airport staff came across to ask if I was feeling alright. I told him that I was afraid that my son may have not caught the flight. 'There is another SAA flight expected any minute,' he said, and I was so relieved that I could feel my knees begin to buckle. He took me across to some chairs

Fly Fishing For Sharks

that were directly in the path of incoming passengers. 'Snubs' as I call Andrew was almost the last person to come through, but as I saw his rueful grin I knew it was going to be a wonderful week.

And there have been other wonderful weeks, other golden threads, but 'living with OCD' is hard, and at times, unbearably sad. That said, what lessons have I learned that could possibly be of any help to you?

1. 'Abort' is not failure.
    Andrew has learned to trust that inner voice that signals the need to withdraw from a situation (as opposed to the tyrannical one that drives his OCD!), because he now knows that each major relapse takes longer to recover from.

2. A psychiatrist (not a GP) and a psychologist make for a whole team.
    Andrew needs the pharmacological base to work out of, but this last year he has benefited enormously from having a professional help him look at the emotional quotient of having OCD, of being depressed, of lost horizons.

3. Take time for yourself
    I have only had two letters published and one of those was about the lesson I learned from Anne Morrow Lindbergh's *Gift from the Sea.* As a mum, a wife, a sister, a daughter, a friend, a professional, etc, there are just so many calls on our time. If you are to be the effective still centre of your particular wheel, take time for yourself. I try to get a couple of hours on the beach every Saturday with my book. I need exercise, film festivals and a summer school top-me-up.

4. Guard your heart; don't be hurt by indifference.
    You will get lots of free 'ice and advice', but trust your instincts, trust what you know of your son. Get a second opinion, and a third if you need. Andrew and I tried to report back to the GP & Serb in Harare; they really weren't interested. I tried to get help from the medical profession in Grahamstown but they were too busy. Psychiatrists on a public holiday in Cape Town were similarly non committal.

5. Remember that you are only human.
    There was a time that I felt so guilty about the fact that I could not give Andrew even one good reason why he should continue with the Sisyphusian struggle that his life had become. Eventually I made an appointment to see one of the sisters at a nearby convent. She didn't judge me. She just looked at me with kind eyes and said 'You are human… God of all people understands… This is your mother's heart speaking.'

6. Let go.
    The hardest part for me, as that Mum Quixote and 'committee of one,' has been to realise that I couldn't 'do' life for Andrew. He has endured; he has survived, and he has done this with the love of a wide support base.

I have already alluded to the many, many people who have played a part in my son's story but I do want to end by thanking especially a co-mum from Alex Park School days, Kay Sayce. It was to her that Andrew sent the first 21 000 words of this manuscript, and it has been her guidance and her encouragement that has brought about this new and positive era in a story that might otherwise never have been told.

Printed in the United Kingdom
by Lightning Source UK Ltd.
133968UK00001B/34-51/P